Prostate Cancer Diet Cookbook For Men Over 40

Sharon Stills

Disclaimer

Please bear in mind that the information in this book is strictly educational. The data presented here is claimed to be credible and trustworthy. The author provides no implied or explicit assurance of accuracy for specific individual instances.

It is important that you consult with a skilled practitioner, such as your doctor, before initiating any diet or lifestyle changes. The information in this book should not be used in place of expert advice or professional assistance.

The author, publisher, and distributor fully disclaim any and all liability, loss, damage, or risk suffered by anybody who relies on the information in this book, whether directly or indirectly.

All intellectual property rights are intact. The content in this book should not be copied in any way, mechanically, electronically, by photocopying, or by any other means available.

CONTENTS

Introduction

As men age, the risk of developing various health conditions increases, and one of the most significant concerns is prostate cancer. Prostate cancer is the second most common cancer among men worldwide, and its prevalence rises sharply after the age of 40. With the increasing incidence of prostate cancer, it is crucial to explore preventative measures and supportive treatments that can help reduce the risk and improve outcomes for those diagnosed. One of the most effective and accessible strategies for managing prostate health is through diet. This book, "Prostate Cancer Diet Cookbook for Men Over 40," aims to provide men with the knowledge and tools they need to make dietary choices that support prostate health, potentially reducing the risk of cancer and improving overall well-being.

Prostate cancer is a major health concern for men, especially those over the age of 40. Statistics show that one in nine men will be diagnosed with prostate cancer at some point in their lives, with the majority of cases occurring in men over 65. However, the risk starts to increase significantly after 40. Factors contributing to this growing concern include:

- **Aging Population**: As life expectancy increases, more men are living into the age range where prostate cancer becomes more common.
- **Lifestyle Factors**: Sedentary lifestyles, poor diet, and obesity are all linked to a higher risk of developing prostate cancer.
- **Genetics**: Family history plays a significant role, and men with close relatives who have had prostate cancer are at a higher risk.

Given these factors, it is essential for men to be proactive about their health, and diet plays a crucial role in this proactive approach.

Numerous studies have shown that diet significantly impacts prostate health. Certain foods can help reduce inflammation, improve immune function, and provide essential nutrients that support the prostate. Conversely, some foods can increase inflammation and contribute to the development of cancerous cells. Key dietary factors that influence prostate health include:

- **Antioxidants**: Found in fruits and vegetables, antioxidants help protect cells from damage.
- **Omega-3 Fatty Acids**: Present in fish and flaxseeds, these fatty acids have anti-inflammatory properties.
- **Vitamins and Minerals**: Nutrients like vitamin D, selenium, and zinc are essential for maintaining prostate health.
- **Fiber**: High-fiber diets are linked to lower cancer risks as they help regulate hormones and remove toxins from the body.

Understanding which foods to include in your diet and which to avoid can have a profound impact on your prostate health. This book provides detailed information on these foods and offers recipes that make it easy to incorporate them into your daily meals.

"Prostate Cancer Diet Cookbook for Men Over 40" is designed to be more than just a collection of recipes. It is a comprehensive guide that addresses the unique dietary needs of men over 40 and provides practical advice on how to create a prostate-healthy eating plan. Here's how this cookbook can help:

- **Educational Resources**: Each chapter includes information on the science behind prostate health and nutrition, helping you understand why certain foods are beneficial.
- **Practical Tips**: From setting up a prostate-healthy kitchen to meal planning and grocery shopping, this book offers practical advice to make healthy eating easy and sustainable.
- **Delicious Recipes**: With a variety of breakfast, lunch, dinner, snack, and dessert recipes, you'll find plenty of options to keep your meals interesting and enjoyable while supporting your prostate health.
- **Lifestyle Integration**: In addition to dietary advice, the book covers other aspects of a healthy lifestyle, such as exercise, stress management, and regular medical check-ups, providing a holistic approach to prostate health.

By following the guidance in this book, men over 40 can take control of their prostate health, reduce their risk of cancer, and improve their overall quality of life. This book empowers you with the knowledge and tools needed to make informed dietary choices that can have a lasting positive impact on your health.

Chapter 1: Understanding Prostate Cancer and Its Impact

What is Prostate Cancer?

Prostate cancer is a type of cancer that occurs in the prostate gland, a small walnut-shaped gland in men that produces seminal fluid, which nourishes and transports sperm. Prostate cancer typically develops slowly and initially remains confined to the prostate gland, where it may not cause serious harm. However, while some types of prostate cancer grow slowly and may need minimal or even no treatment, other types are aggressive and can spread quickly.

Types of Prostate Cancer:
1. **Adenocarcinomas:** The most common type, originating in the gland cells.
2. **Small Cell Carcinomas:** A rare and aggressive form.
3. **Neuroendocrine Tumors:** Another rare form that can be aggressive.
4. **Transitional Cell Carcinomas:** Typically starts in the bladder and spreads to the prostate.

Stages of Prostate Cancer:
1. **Stage I:** Cancer is small and only in the prostate.
2. **Stage II:** Cancer is larger but still confined to the prostate.
3. **Stage III:** Cancer has spread to nearby tissues.
4. **Stage IV:** Cancer has spread to other parts of the body.

Understanding the nature of prostate cancer, including its types and stages, is crucial for grasping the significance of early detection and treatment strategies.

Risk Factors and Symptoms

Prostate cancer risk factors can be categorized into those that cannot be controlled and those that can be influenced by lifestyle choices.

Uncontrollable Risk Factors:
1. **Age:** Risk increases significantly after age 50.
2. **Race/Ethnicity:** African-American men have a higher risk of developing and dying from prostate cancer.
3. **Family History:** A family history of prostate cancer increases risk.
4. **Genetic Mutations:** Certain genetic changes, such as mutations in the BRCA1 and BRCA2 genes, can increase risk.

Controllable Risk Factors:
1. **Diet:** Diets high in red meat and high-fat dairy products and low in fruits and vegetables may increase risk.

2. **Obesity:** Obesity has been linked to a higher risk of prostate cancer and more aggressive forms of the disease.
3. **Smoking:** Smoking is associated with a higher risk of death from prostate cancer.

Symptoms of Prostate Cancer:
In its early stages, prostate cancer may not cause noticeable symptoms. However, as it advances, it may cause:
1. **Urinary Symptoms:**
   - Difficulty starting or stopping urination.
   - Weak or interrupted flow of urine.
   - Frequent urination, especially at night.
   - Pain or burning sensation during urination.
2. **Sexual Dysfunction:**
   - Difficulty achieving an erection.
   - Painful ejaculation.
3. **Advanced Symptoms:**
   - Blood in urine or semen.
   - Pain in the back, hips, or pelvis.
   - Unexplained weight loss and fatigue.

Recognizing these symptoms and seeking medical advice promptly can lead to earlier detection and more effective treatment.

The Importance of Early Detection

Early detection of prostate cancer is crucial because it significantly increases the chances of successful treatment and reduces the likelihood of the cancer spreading. Several methods are used for early detection:
1. **Prostate-Specific Antigen (PSA) Test:** Measures the level of PSA in the blood. Elevated levels may indicate prostate cancer, but can also be due to other prostate conditions.
2. **Digital Rectal Exam (DRE):** A healthcare provider inserts a gloved, lubricated finger into the rectum to check the prostate for abnormalities.
3. **Biopsy:** If PSA or DRE results are abnormal, a biopsy may be performed to confirm the presence of cancer cells.

Benefits of Early Detection:
1. **More Treatment Options:** Early-stage cancer can often be treated more effectively with a wider range of options.
2. **Better Outcomes:** The survival rate for prostate cancer detected at an early stage is very high.
3. **Less Aggressive Treatment:** Early detection may allow for less aggressive treatments, reducing the risk of side effects.

The Role of Diet in Prevention and Management

Diet plays a pivotal role in both the prevention and management of prostate cancer. Research indicates that certain dietary patterns can reduce the risk of developing prostate cancer and improve outcomes for those already diagnosed.

Preventive Dietary Strategies:
1. **Fruits and Vegetables:** Rich in antioxidants, vitamins, and minerals, they help protect cells from damage. Cruciferous vegetables (like broccoli and cauliflower) and tomatoes (rich in lycopene) are particularly beneficial.
2. **Healthy Fats:** Omega-3 fatty acids found in fish (like salmon and mackerel) have anti-inflammatory properties that may reduce cancer risk. Avoid trans fats and reduce saturated fat intake.
3. **Whole Grains:** High in fiber, whole grains can help regulate hormones and reduce cancer risk. Examples include brown rice, oatmeal, and whole wheat bread.
4. **Green Tea:** Contains catechins, which are antioxidants that may protect against cancer cell development.

Dietary Management for Prostate Cancer Patients:
1. **Low-Fat Diet:** Reducing fat intake, particularly from animal sources, can help manage weight and lower the risk of cancer progression.
2. **Plant-Based Diet:** Emphasizing plant-based foods over animal products can provide essential nutrients and lower inflammation.
3. **Soy Products:** Soy contains phytoestrogens that may help regulate hormone levels and reduce cancer risk.
4. **Limit Processed Foods:** Processed foods often contain unhealthy fats, sugars, and additives that can contribute to cancer risk and overall poor health.

Integrating Diet into Lifestyle:
1. **Consistency:** Making dietary changes a regular part of daily life can help maintain prostate health in the long term.
2. **Education:** Learning about which foods are beneficial and how to prepare them can empower men to make healthier choices.
3. **Support:** Engaging with community resources, support groups, and healthcare providers can provide encouragement and practical advice.

By adopting a prostate-healthy diet, men can take a proactive role in reducing their risk of prostate cancer and managing their health if diagnosed. This chapter underscores the critical connection between diet and prostate health, setting the stage for the practical guidance and recipes provided in the subsequent chapters of this book.

Chapter 2: The Prostate-Healthy Diet

Key Nutrients for Prostate Health

Proper nutrition plays a vital role in maintaining prostate health and reducing the risk of prostate cancer. Certain nutrients have been identified as particularly beneficial for the prostate:

1. **Lycopene**:
   - **Sources**: Tomatoes, watermelon, pink grapefruit, and papaya.
   - **Benefits**: Lycopene is a powerful antioxidant that helps protect cells from damage. Studies have shown that a diet rich in lycopene can reduce the risk of prostate cancer and may slow the progression of existing cancer.
2. **Omega-3 Fatty Acids**:
   - **Sources**: Fatty fish (salmon, mackerel, sardines), flaxseeds, chia seeds, and walnuts.
   - **Benefits**: Omega-3 fatty acids have anti-inflammatory properties that help reduce inflammation, which is linked to cancer development. These fatty acids also support overall heart health, which is important for men over 40.
3. **Vitamin D**:
   - **Sources**: Sunlight exposure, fortified foods (milk, orange juice), fatty fish, and supplements.
   - **Benefits**: Vitamin D plays a role in regulating cell growth and differentiation. Adequate levels of vitamin D are associated with a lower risk of prostate cancer.
4. **Selenium**:
   - **Sources**: Brazil nuts, seafood, eggs, and grains.
   - **Benefits**: Selenium is a trace mineral with antioxidant properties. It has been shown to help protect against cancer by preventing cell damage and supporting the immune system.
5. **Zinc**:
   - **Sources**: Meat, shellfish, legumes, seeds, and nuts.
   - **Benefits**: Zinc is crucial for maintaining a healthy immune system and has been linked to prostate health. It plays a role in the regulation of prostate growth and function.
6. **Cruciferous Vegetables**:
   - **Sources**: Broccoli, cauliflower, Brussels sprouts, kale, and cabbage.
   - **Benefits**: These vegetables contain sulforaphane, a compound that has been shown to help protect against cancer by promoting the elimination of potential carcinogens from the body.
7. **Antioxidants**:
   - **Sources**: Fruits and vegetables, particularly berries, citrus fruits, leafy greens, and nuts.
   - **Benefits**: Antioxidants neutralize free radicals, reducing oxidative stress and DNA damage that can lead to cancer.

Foods to Include in Your Diet

Incorporating a variety of nutrient-rich foods into your diet can support prostate health and reduce the risk of prostate cancer. Here are some key foods to include:

1. **Tomatoes**:
   - Rich in lycopene, which has been shown to reduce prostate cancer risk.
   - Cooking tomatoes increases the bioavailability of lycopene.
2. **Fatty Fish**:
   - Sources include salmon, mackerel, and sardines, which are high in omega-3 fatty acids.
   - Aim for at least two servings per week.
3. **Berries**:
   - Blueberries, strawberries, raspberries, and blackberries are high in antioxidants.
   - These fruits help reduce oxidative stress and inflammation.
4. **Green Tea**:
   - Contains catechins, antioxidants that may protect against cancer cell development.
   - Regular consumption can support overall health.
5. **Nuts and Seeds**:
   - Walnuts, flaxseeds, and chia seeds are excellent sources of omega-3 fatty acids and other beneficial nutrients.
   - Brazil nuts provide a significant amount of selenium.
6. **Legumes and Soy Products**:
   - Beans, lentils, tofu, and tempeh are rich in fiber, protein, and phytoestrogens, which may help regulate hormones.
   - Soy products have been linked to a reduced risk of prostate cancer.
7. **Whole Grains**:
   - Brown rice, quinoa, oatmeal, and whole wheat products are high in fiber, which helps in regulating hormone levels and maintaining a healthy weight.
   - Whole grains also provide essential vitamins and minerals.
8. **Cruciferous Vegetables**:
   - Broccoli, cauliflower, Brussels sprouts, and kale are high in sulforaphane.
   - Regular consumption can help detoxify the body and protect against cancer.
9. **Citrus Fruits**:
   - Oranges, lemons, limes, and grapefruits are rich in vitamin C and other antioxidants.
   - These fruits support the immune system and overall health.

Foods to Avoid

Just as important as the foods to include are the foods to avoid, which can increase the risk of prostate cancer and other health issues:

1. **Red and Processed Meats**:
   - High consumption of red meats (beef, pork, lamb) and processed meats (sausages, hot dogs, bacon) has been linked to an increased risk of prostate cancer.
   - These meats contain carcinogens that form during cooking at high temperatures.
2. **High-Fat Dairy Products**:
   - Whole milk, cheese, and butter are high in saturated fats, which can promote inflammation and cancer growth.
   - Opt for low-fat or plant-based dairy alternatives.
3. **Fried Foods**:
   - Foods cooked in unhealthy oils and at high temperatures can contain harmful compounds.
   - These compounds can increase inflammation and the risk of cancer.
4. **Sugary Foods and Beverages**:
   - High consumption of sugary drinks and snacks can lead to obesity, a risk factor for prostate cancer.
   - These foods also contribute to inflammation and insulin resistance.
5. **Alcohol**:
   - Excessive alcohol consumption can increase the risk of prostate cancer.
   - Limit alcohol intake to moderate levels (up to one drink per day).
6. **Refined Grains**:
   - White bread, white rice, and other refined grains lack fiber and essential nutrients.
   - These foods can cause spikes in blood sugar levels and contribute to weight gain.

The Science Behind Prostate-Healthy Foods

The benefits of prostate-healthy foods are supported by a growing body of scientific research. Understanding the mechanisms behind these benefits can help underscore the importance of dietary choices:

1. **Antioxidants and Free Radicals**:
   - Free radicals are unstable molecules that can damage cells and DNA, leading to cancer.
   - Antioxidants neutralize free radicals, reducing oxidative stress and the risk of cancer development.
2. **Anti-Inflammatory Properties**:
   - Chronic inflammation is linked to cancer progression.
   - Omega-3 fatty acids and certain plant compounds (e.g., sulforaphane in cruciferous vegetables) have anti-inflammatory effects that help reduce this risk.

3. **Hormonal Regulation**:
   - Prostate cancer is influenced by hormones, particularly testosterone and its derivative, dihydrotestosterone (DHT).
   - Foods rich in phytoestrogens (soy products) and fiber help regulate hormone levels, reducing cancer risk.
4. **Detoxification**:
   - Certain foods, like cruciferous vegetables, support the body's natural detoxification processes.
   - Sulforaphane promotes the elimination of potential carcinogens from the body.
5. **Immune System Support**:
   - A strong immune system helps detect and destroy cancer cells before they proliferate.
   - Nutrient-rich foods, particularly those high in vitamins C and D, zinc, and selenium, support immune function.
6. **Cell Growth and Repair**:
   - Nutrients like vitamin D and omega-3 fatty acids play roles in regulating cell growth and repair.
   - Proper cell function and regulation are crucial in preventing the uncontrolled growth characteristic of cancer.

In summary, a prostate-healthy diet rich in specific nutrients and foods can play a significant role in preventing prostate cancer and supporting overall prostate health. By understanding the benefits of key nutrients and making informed dietary choices, men over 40 can proactively manage their health and reduce their risk of prostate-related issues.

Chapter 3: Setting Up Your Prostate-Healthy Kitchen

Creating a kitchen that supports a prostate-healthy diet involves more than just selecting the right foods. It requires thoughtful organization, planning, and equipping your kitchen with the right tools and ingredients. This chapter provides a comprehensive guide to setting up a prostate-healthy kitchen, ensuring you have everything you need to prepare nutritious and delicious meals.

Essential Kitchen Tools and Equipment

Having the right tools and equipment in your kitchen can make preparing prostate-healthy meals easier and more enjoyable. Here are some essentials:

1. **High-Quality Knives**: Invest in a good set of knives, including a chef's knife, paring knife, and serrated knife. Sharp knives make chopping fruits, vegetables, and other ingredients safer and more efficient.
2. **Cutting Boards**: Use separate cutting boards for meat and vegetables to avoid cross-contamination. Choose durable, easy-to-clean materials like bamboo or plastic.
3. **Blender**: A high-powered blender is essential for making smoothies, soups, and sauces. It can also be used to blend nuts and seeds into nut butters or to make healthy dressings.
4. **Food Processor**: This versatile tool can chop, slice, shred, and puree ingredients, making meal prep faster and more efficient.
5. **Steamer Basket**: Steaming is a healthy cooking method that preserves the nutrients in vegetables. A steamer basket can be used in any pot and is an affordable addition to your kitchen.
6. **Non-Stick Cookware**: Invest in a set of non-stick pans for cooking with minimal oil. This is especially useful for reducing the intake of unhealthy fats.
7. **Measuring Cups and Spoons**: Accurate measurements are crucial for following recipes and maintaining portion control.
8. **Mixing Bowls**: A set of mixing bowls in various sizes is essential for preparing and mixing ingredients.
9. **Baking Sheets and Pans**: These are necessary for baking vegetables, proteins, and healthy snacks.
10. **Storage Containers**: Invest in a variety of airtight containers for storing prepped ingredients, leftovers, and batch-cooked meals. Glass containers are a great option for avoiding plastic chemicals.
11. **Spiralizer**: This tool is great for making vegetable noodles from zucchini, carrots, and other veggies, providing a low-carb alternative to pasta.

Stocking Your Pantry with Prostate-Healthy Staples

A well-stocked pantry ensures that you always have the ingredients needed to prepare healthy meals, even on busy days. Here are key prostate-healthy staples to keep on hand:

1. **Whole Grains**: Brown rice, quinoa, barley, whole wheat pasta, and oats. These provide fiber, vitamins, and minerals.
2. **Legumes**: Canned or dried beans (black beans, chickpeas, lentils) are excellent sources of plant-based protein and fiber.
3. **Nuts and Seeds**: Almonds, walnuts, flaxseeds, chia seeds, and pumpkin seeds are rich in healthy fats, protein, and fiber.
4. **Healthy Oils**: Olive oil, avocado oil, and flaxseed oil are good for cooking and dressings due to their beneficial fats.
5. **Spices and Herbs**: Turmeric, ginger, garlic, basil, oregano, and rosemary not only add flavor but also provide anti-inflammatory benefits.
6. **Canned Tomatoes**: Use these for sauces, soups, and stews. They are a convenient source of lycopene.
7. **Frozen Fruits and Vegetables**: Keep a variety of frozen produce for smoothies, soups, and side dishes.
8. **Whole Grain Flours**: Whole wheat flour, almond flour, and oat flour for baking healthier versions of your favorite recipes.
9. **Low-Sodium Broths**: Vegetable, chicken, or beef broths for soups and stews.
10. **Nut Butters**: Almond butter, peanut butter, and cashew butter are great for snacks and adding to smoothies.
11. **Dried Fruits**: Raisins, apricots, and cranberries can be used in salads, snacks, and baking for added sweetness and nutrients.

Meal Planning Tips for Busy Men Over 40

Effective meal planning can save time, reduce stress, and ensure that you maintain a prostate-healthy diet even with a busy schedule. Here are some tips:

1. **Plan Ahead**: Take some time each week to plan your meals. This helps ensure that you have all the necessary ingredients and reduces the likelihood of unhealthy, last-minute food choices.
2. **Batch Cooking**: Prepare large quantities of staples like grains, beans, and roasted vegetables. Store them in the refrigerator or freezer to use throughout the week.
3. **Prep Ingredients**: Wash and chop vegetables, marinate proteins, and prepare snacks in advance. This reduces the time needed to cook meals on busy days.
4. **Use a Meal Planner**: Utilize a meal planning app or a simple notebook to track your meals for the week. Include breakfast, lunch, dinner, and snacks.
5. **Cook Once, Eat Twice**: Make double portions of dinner and pack the leftovers for lunch the next day. This saves time and ensures you have a healthy meal ready to go.
6. **Keep it Simple**: Focus on simple recipes with minimal ingredients. This makes cooking less daunting and more manageable.
7. **Incorporate Variety**: Rotate different types of proteins, grains, and vegetables to keep meals interesting and ensure a wide range of nutrients.

8. **Healthy Snacks**: Prepare healthy snacks like cut vegetables, hummus, nuts, and fruits to have on hand for when hunger strikes between meals.

Shopping List for Prostate Health

Having a well-prepared shopping list ensures that you purchase everything needed to maintain a prostate-healthy diet. Here's a sample shopping list to get you started:

Produce:

- Tomatoes
- Leafy greens (spinach, kale, Swiss chard)
- Cruciferous vegetables (broccoli, cauliflower, Brussels sprouts)
- Berries (blueberries, strawberries, raspberries)
- Citrus fruits (oranges, lemons, limes, grapefruits)
- Apples and pears
- Avocados
- Garlic and onions
- Carrots and bell peppers
- Zucchini and squash
- Mushrooms

Proteins:

- Lean meats (chicken, turkey)
- Fatty fish (salmon, mackerel, sardines)
- Eggs
- Tofu and tempeh
- Legumes (black beans, chickpeas, lentils)

Grains and Cereals:

- Brown rice
- Quinoa
- Oats
- Whole wheat bread and pasta
- Barley

Nuts and Seeds:

- Almonds and walnuts
- Chia seeds and flaxseeds
- Pumpkin seeds and sunflower seeds

Dairy and Alternatives:

- Low-fat or plant-based milk (almond milk, soy milk)
- Low-fat yogurt or plant-based yogurt
- Low-fat cheese or plant-based cheese

Pantry Staples:
- Olive oil and avocado oil
- Low-sodium vegetable, chicken, or beef broth
- Canned tomatoes
- Nut butters (almond butter, peanut butter)
- Whole grain flours (whole wheat flour, almond flour)
- Dried fruits (raisins, apricots, cranberries)

Spices and Herbs:
- Turmeric
- Ginger
- Garlic powder
- Basil
- Oregano
- Rosemary
- Black pepper
- Cinnamon

Beverages:
- Green tea
- Herbal teas
- Unsweetened fruit juices

By setting up your kitchen with the right tools, stocking it with prostate-healthy staples, and planning your meals effectively, you can make it easier to maintain a diet that supports prostate health.

Breakfast

Tomato and Spinach Omelette

Total Time: 15 minutes
Number of Servings: 1

Ingredients:
- 2 large eggs
- 1/4 cup fresh spinach, chopped
- 1/4 cup cherry tomatoes, halved
- 1 tablespoon olive oil
- Salt and pepper to taste
- 1 tablespoon grated Parmesan cheese (optional)

Directions:
1. In a bowl, beat the eggs with a pinch of salt and pepper.
2. Heat olive oil in a non-stick skillet over medium heat.
3. Add the chopped spinach and cook until wilted, about 2 minutes.
4. Add the cherry tomatoes and cook for another 2 minutes.
5. Pour the beaten eggs over the spinach and tomatoes. Tilt the pan to spread the eggs evenly.
6. Cook until the edges start to set, then gently lift the edges to let the uncooked eggs flow underneath.
7. Once the eggs are mostly set, sprinkle with Parmesan cheese, if using.
8. Fold the omelette in half and cook for another minute.
9. Serve hot.

Nutritional Information (per serving):
- Calories: 200
- Protein: 14g
- Fat: 14g
- Carbohydrates: 4g
- Fiber: 1g

Berry and Chia Seed Overnight Oats

Total Time: 10 minutes (plus overnight soaking)
Number of Servings: 1

Ingredients:
- 1/2 cup rolled oats

- 1/2 cup unsweetened almond milk
- 1/4 cup mixed berries (blueberries, strawberries, raspberries)
- 1 tablespoon chia seeds
- 1 teaspoon honey or maple syrup (optional)

Directions:
1. In a mason jar or bowl, combine the rolled oats, almond milk, chia seeds, and honey/maple syrup.
2. Stir well to combine.
3. Top with mixed berries.
4. Cover and refrigerate overnight (or at least 4 hours).
5. In the morning, stir the oats and enjoy cold or heated.

Nutritional Information (per serving):
- Calories: 250
- Protein: 7g
- Fat: 7g
- Carbohydrates: 42g
- Fiber: 10g

Avocado Toast with Whole Grain Bread

Total Time: 10 minutes
Number of Servings: 1

Ingredients:
- 1 slice whole grain bread
- 1/2 ripe avocado
- Salt and pepper to taste
- Red pepper flakes (optional)
- 1 teaspoon lemon juice (optional)

Directions:
1. Toast the whole grain bread to your liking.
2. While the bread is toasting, mash the avocado in a bowl with a fork.
3. Add salt, pepper, and lemon juice to the mashed avocado and mix well.
4. Spread the mashed avocado on the toasted bread.
5. Sprinkle with red pepper flakes, if desired.
6. Serve immediately.

Nutritional Information (per serving):
- Calories: 220
- Protein: 5g
- Fat: 16g

- Carbohydrates: 20g
- Fiber: 8g

Quinoa Breakfast Bowl with Berries and Nuts

Total Time: 20 minutes
Number of Servings: 2

Ingredients:
- 1 cup cooked quinoa
- 1/2 cup mixed berries (blueberries, strawberries, raspberries)
- 2 tablespoons chopped nuts (almonds, walnuts, or pecans)
- 1 tablespoon chia seeds
- 1 cup unsweetened almond milk
- 1 teaspoon honey or maple syrup (optional)
- 1/2 teaspoon cinnamon (optional)

Directions:
1. In a medium-sized bowl, combine the cooked quinoa and almond milk.
2. Stir in the chia seeds, honey/maple syrup, and cinnamon, if using.
3. Divide the mixture into two serving bowls.
4. Top each bowl with mixed berries and chopped nuts.
5. Serve immediately.

Nutritional Information (per serving):
- Calories: 300
- Protein: 9g
- Fat: 12g
- Carbohydrates: 42g
- Fiber: 8g

Greek Yogurt with Flaxseeds and Honey

Total Time: 5 minutes
Number of Servings: 1

Ingredients:
- 1 cup plain Greek yogurt
- 1 tablespoon ground flaxseeds
- 1 teaspoon honey
- 1/4 cup fresh berries (optional)

Directions:
1. In a bowl, add the Greek yogurt.
2. Sprinkle the ground flaxseeds over the yogurt.
3. Drizzle with honey.
4. Top with fresh berries, if desired.
5. Stir gently to combine and serve immediately.

Nutritional Information (per serving):
- Calories: 180
- Protein: 15g
- Fat: 5g
- Carbohydrates: 20g
- Fiber: 4g

Green Smoothie Bowl with Spinach, Banana, and Almond Milk

Total Time: 10 minutes
Number of Servings: 1

Ingredients:
- 1 ripe banana, frozen
- 1 cup fresh spinach
- 1/2 cup unsweetened almond milk
- 1 tablespoon chia seeds
- 1 tablespoon almond butter
- Fresh berries and sliced banana for topping
- Granola or nuts for topping (optional)

Directions:
1. In a blender, combine the frozen banana, fresh spinach, almond milk, chia seeds, and almond butter.
2. Blend until smooth and creamy.
3. Pour the smoothie into a bowl.
4. Top with fresh berries, sliced banana, and granola or nuts if desired.
5. Serve immediately and enjoy!

Nutritional Information (per serving):
- Calories: 320
- Protein: 8g
- Fat: 14g
- Carbohydrates: 45g
- Fiber: 12g

Steel-Cut Oats with Walnuts and Blueberries

Total Time: 30 minutes
Number of Servings: 2

Ingredients:
- 1 cup steel-cut oats
- 2 cups water
- 1 cup unsweetened almond milk
- 1/4 cup chopped walnuts
- 1/2 cup fresh blueberries
- 1 tablespoon honey or maple syrup (optional)
- Pinch of cinnamon (optional)

Directions:
1. In a saucepan, bring the water to a boil.
2. Stir in the steel-cut oats and reduce heat to low.
3. Simmer for 20-25 minutes, stirring occasionally, until oats are tender and creamy.
4. Stir in the almond milk and cook for an additional 5 minutes.
5. Remove from heat and stir in the chopped walnuts, fresh blueberries, honey/maple syrup, and cinnamon if desired.
6. Divide into serving bowls and serve hot.

Nutritional Information (per serving):
- Calories: 280
- Protein: 9g
- Fat: 9g
- Carbohydrates: 44g
- Fiber: 7g

Whole Grain Pancakes with Fresh Berries

Total Time: 20 minutes
Number of Servings: 2

Ingredients:
- 1 cup whole grain pancake mix
- 3/4 cup unsweetened almond milk
- 1 egg
- 1 tablespoon olive oil or melted coconut oil
- 1 cup fresh berries (blueberries, strawberries, raspberries)
- Maple syrup for serving (optional)

Directions:
1. In a mixing bowl, whisk together the pancake mix, almond milk, egg, and olive oil until smooth.
2. Heat a non-stick skillet or griddle over medium heat and lightly grease with oil or cooking spray.
3. Pour about 1/4 cup of batter onto the skillet for each pancake.
4. Cook for 2-3 minutes on each side, until golden brown and cooked through.
5. Stack the pancakes on serving plates and top with fresh berries.
6. Serve warm with maple syrup if desired.

Nutritional Information (per serving):
- Calories: 300
- Protein: 8g
- Fat: 10g
- Carbohydrates: 45g
- Fiber: 7g

Scrambled Eggs with Turmeric and Kale

Total Time: 15 minutes
Number of Servings: 2

Ingredients:
- 4 large eggs
- 1 cup chopped kale
- 1/2 teaspoon ground turmeric
- Salt and pepper to taste
- 1 tablespoon olive oil or butter
- Optional: grated cheese for topping

Directions:
1. In a bowl, whisk together the eggs, ground turmeric, salt, and pepper until well combined.
2. Heat olive oil or butter in a skillet over medium heat.
3. Add the chopped kale to the skillet and cook for 2-3 minutes until wilted.
4. Pour the whisked eggs over the kale and let cook for 1-2 minutes until the edges start to set.
5. Use a spatula to gently scramble the eggs until cooked through.
6. Remove from heat and serve hot.
7. Optionally, sprinkle grated cheese on top before serving.

Nutritional Information (per serving):
- Calories: 200
- Protein: 14g

- Fat: 14g
- Carbohydrates: 4g
- Fiber: 1g

Chia Seed Pudding with Almond Milk and Fresh Fruit

Total Time: 5 minutes (plus 4 hours chilling time)
Number of Servings: 2

Ingredients:
- 1/4 cup chia seeds
- 1 cup unsweetened almond milk
- 1 tablespoon honey or maple syrup
- 1/2 teaspoon vanilla extract
- Fresh fruit for topping (strawberries, blueberries, kiwi)

Directions:
1. In a bowl, mix together the chia seeds, almond milk, honey/maple syrup, and vanilla extract.
2. Stir well until combined.
3. Cover the bowl and refrigerate for at least 4 hours or overnight, until the mixture thickens into a pudding-like consistency.
4. Divide the chia seed pudding into serving bowls.
5. Top with fresh fruit before serving.

Nutritional Information (per serving):
- Calories: 150
- Protein: 4g
- Fat: 8g
- Carbohydrates: 16g
- Fiber: 9g

Cottage Cheese with Pineapple and Flaxseeds

Total Time: 5 minutes
Number of Servings: 1

Ingredients:
- 1/2 cup cottage cheese
- 1/2 cup fresh pineapple chunks
- 1 tablespoon ground flaxseeds

Directions:

1. In a bowl, combine the cottage cheese and fresh pineapple chunks.
2. Sprinkle ground flaxseeds on top.
3. Mix well and enjoy.

Nutritional Information (per serving):

- Calories: 200
- Protein: 20g
- Fat: 6g
- Carbohydrates: 18g
- Fiber: 3g

Sweet Potato and Black Bean Breakfast Burrito

Total Time: 30 minutes
Number of Servings: 2

Ingredients:

- 2 large whole wheat tortillas
- 1 medium sweet potato, diced
- 1/2 cup canned black beans, drained and rinsed
- 1/2 bell pepper, diced
- 2 eggs, scrambled
- 1/4 cup shredded cheddar cheese
- Salt and pepper to taste
- Optional toppings: salsa, avocado, Greek yogurt

Directions:

1. Preheat the oven to 400°F (200°C).
2. Place diced sweet potato on a baking sheet, drizzle with olive oil, and season with salt and pepper. Roast for 20-25 minutes until tender.
3. In a skillet, sauté the bell pepper until softened.
4. Add the black beans and cooked sweet potato to the skillet. Cook until heated through.
5. In another skillet, scramble the eggs until cooked.
6. Warm the tortillas in a dry skillet or microwave.
7. Divide the sweet potato and black bean mixture, scrambled eggs, and shredded cheese between the tortillas.
8. Roll up the tortillas to form burritos.
9. Serve with optional toppings like salsa, avocado, or Greek yogurt.

Nutritional Information (per serving):

- Calories: 380
- Protein: 18g
- Fat: 14g

- Carbohydrates: 50g
- Fiber: 10g

Mushroom and Tomato Frittata

Total Time: 25 minutes
Number of Servings: 4

Ingredients:
- 8 large eggs
- 1 cup sliced mushrooms
- 1 cup cherry tomatoes, halved
- 1/2 cup diced onion
- 1/4 cup chopped fresh parsley
- 1/4 cup grated Parmesan cheese
- Salt and pepper to taste
- 1 tablespoon olive oil

Directions:
1. Preheat the broiler in your oven.
2. In a large oven-safe skillet, heat olive oil over medium heat.
3. Add diced onion and sliced mushrooms to the skillet. Cook until softened, about 5 minutes.
4. In a bowl, whisk together the eggs, chopped parsley, grated Parmesan cheese, salt, and pepper.
5. Pour the egg mixture over the vegetables in the skillet. Stir gently to distribute the ingredients evenly.
6. Cook on the stovetop for 5-7 minutes until the edges start to set.
7. Place the skillet under the broiler for 3-5 minutes until the top is set and lightly golden.
8. Remove from the oven and let cool slightly before slicing into wedges.
9. Serve warm.

Nutritional Information (per serving):
- Calories: 180
- Protein: 13g
- Fat: 12g
- Carbohydrates: 5g
- Fiber: 1g

Whole Grain Muffins with Apple and Carrot

Total Time: 35 minutes
Number of Servings: 12 muffins

Ingredients:
- 1 1/2 cups whole wheat flour
- 1 teaspoon baking powder
- 1/2 teaspoon baking soda
- 1/2 teaspoon ground cinnamon
- 1/4 teaspoon ground nutmeg
- 1/4 teaspoon salt
- 2 large eggs
- 1/2 cup unsweetened applesauce
- 1/4 cup honey or maple syrup
- 1/4 cup olive oil
- 1 cup grated apple
- 1/2 cup grated carrot
- 1/4 cup chopped walnuts or pecans (optional)

Directions:
1. Preheat the oven to 350°F (175°C). Line a muffin tin with paper liners or grease with cooking spray.
2. In a large bowl, whisk together the whole wheat flour, baking powder, baking soda, cinnamon, nutmeg, and salt.
3. In another bowl, beat the eggs and then stir in the applesauce, honey/maple syrup, and olive oil until well combined.
4. Pour the wet ingredients into the dry ingredients and mix until just combined.
5. Fold in the grated apple, grated carrot, and chopped nuts (if using).
6. Divide the batter evenly among the muffin cups, filling each about 3/4 full.
7. Bake for 20-25 minutes, or until a toothpick inserted into the center comes out clean.
8. Allow the muffins to cool in the pan for 5 minutes, then transfer to a wire rack to cool completely.
9. Enjoy warm or store in an airtight container for later.

Nutritional Information (per serving - 1 muffin):
- Calories: 140
- Protein: 3g
- Fat: 6g
- Carbohydrates: 19g
- Fiber: 2g

Smoothie Bowl with Spinach, Avocado, and Pumpkin Seeds

Total Time: 10 minutes
Number of Servings: 1

Ingredients:
- 1 ripe banana
- 1/2 ripe avocado
- 1 cup fresh spinach
- 1/2 cup unsweetened almond milk
- 2 tablespoons pumpkin seeds
- Optional toppings: sliced banana, berries, granola, honey

Directions:
1. In a blender, combine the ripe banana, ripe avocado, fresh spinach, and unsweetened almond milk.
2. Blend until smooth and creamy.
3. Pour the smoothie into a bowl.
4. Top with pumpkin seeds and any optional toppings of your choice.
5. Serve immediately and enjoy!

Nutritional Information (per serving):
- Calories: 350
- Protein: 10g
- Fat: 20g
- Carbohydrates: 40g
- Fiber: 12g

Lunch

Grilled Chicken and Quinoa Salad with Lemon Dressing

Total Time: 30 minutes
Number of Servings: 4

Ingredients:
- 2 boneless, skinless chicken breasts
- 1 cup quinoa
- 2 cups water or chicken broth
- 2 cups mixed salad greens
- 1 cup cherry tomatoes, halved
- 1/2 cucumber, sliced
- 1/4 cup red onion, thinly sliced
- 1/4 cup feta cheese, crumbled
- 2 tablespoons chopped fresh parsley
- Salt and pepper to taste

Lemon Dressing:
- 1/4 cup olive oil
- 2 tablespoons fresh lemon juice
- 1 teaspoon Dijon mustard
- 1 teaspoon honey or maple syrup
- Salt and pepper to taste

Directions:
1. Season the chicken breasts with salt and pepper. Grill or pan-sear until cooked through, about 6-8 minutes per side. Let cool, then slice into strips.
2. Rinse the quinoa under cold water. In a saucepan, bring the water or chicken broth to a boil. Add the quinoa, reduce heat to low, cover, and simmer for 15 minutes. Remove from heat and let sit for 5 minutes. Fluff with a fork.
3. In a large mixing bowl, combine the cooked quinoa, mixed salad greens, cherry tomatoes, cucumber, red onion, feta cheese, and chopped parsley.
4. In a small bowl, whisk together the ingredients for the lemon dressing until well combined.
5. Pour the lemon dressing over the salad and toss to coat evenly.
6. Divide the salad into serving bowls and top with sliced grilled chicken.
7. Serve immediately and enjoy!

Nutritional Information (per serving):
- Calories: 380
- Protein: 25g

- Fat: 16g
- Carbohydrates: 35g
- Fiber: 5g

Lentil and Vegetable Soup

Total Time: 45 minutes
Number of Servings: 6

Ingredients:
- 1 cup dried lentils, rinsed and drained
- 1 tablespoon olive oil
- 1 onion, diced
- 2 carrots, diced
- 2 celery stalks, diced
- 3 cloves garlic, minced
- 1 teaspoon ground cumin
- 1 teaspoon ground coriander
- 1/2 teaspoon smoked paprika
- 6 cups vegetable or chicken broth
- 1 can (14 oz) diced tomatoes
- 2 cups chopped spinach or kale
- Salt and pepper to taste
- Fresh parsley for garnish (optional)

Directions:
1. In a large pot, heat olive oil over medium heat. Add the diced onion, carrots, and celery. Cook until softened, about 5 minutes.
2. Add the minced garlic, ground cumin, ground coriander, and smoked paprika. Cook for another 1-2 minutes until fragrant.
3. Add the rinsed lentils, broth, and diced tomatoes to the pot. Bring to a boil, then reduce heat to low and simmer for 25-30 minutes, until lentils are tender.
4. Stir in the chopped spinach or kale and cook for an additional 5 minutes until wilted.
5. Season with salt and pepper to taste.
6. Ladle the soup into serving bowls, garnish with fresh parsley if desired, and serve hot.

Nutritional Information (per serving):
- Calories: 220
- Protein: 12g
- Fat: 3g
- Carbohydrates: 38g
- Fiber: 10g

Spinach and Tomato Whole Wheat Wrap

Total Time: 10 minutes
Number of Servings: 1

Ingredients:
- 1 whole wheat tortilla
- 1/2 cup fresh spinach leaves
- 1/4 cup cherry tomatoes, halved
- 1/4 cup shredded carrots
- 2 tablespoons hummus
- Salt and pepper to taste

Directions:
1. Lay the whole wheat tortilla flat on a clean surface.
2. Spread hummus evenly over the tortilla.
3. Layer fresh spinach leaves, cherry tomatoes, and shredded carrots on top of the hummus.
4. Season with salt and pepper to taste.
5. Roll up the tortilla tightly.
6. Cut the wrap in half diagonally and serve immediately.

Nutritional Information (per serving):
- Calories: 250
- Protein: 9g
- Fat: 8g
- Carbohydrates: 35g
- Fiber: 9g

Turkey and Avocado Whole Grain Sandwich

Total Time: 10 minutes
Number of Servings: 1

Ingredients:
- 2 slices whole grain bread
- 2-3 slices deli turkey breast
- 1/4 avocado, sliced
- 1/4 cup mixed salad greens
- 1 tablespoon Dijon mustard
- Salt and pepper to taste

Directions:

1. Toast the whole grain bread to your liking.
2. Spread Dijon mustard on one slice of bread.
3. Layer deli turkey breast, sliced avocado, and mixed salad greens on top of the mustard.
4. Season with salt and pepper to taste.
5. Top with the second slice of bread to form a sandwich.
6. Slice in half diagonally and serve immediately.

Nutritional Information (per serving):

- Calories: 300
- Protein: 20g
- Fat: 12g
- Carbohydrates: 28g
- Fiber: 8g

Chickpea and Spinach Curry

Total Time: 30 minutes
Number of Servings: 4

Ingredients:

- 2 tablespoons olive oil
- 1 onion, finely chopped
- 3 cloves garlic, minced
- 1 tablespoon grated ginger
- 1 teaspoon ground cumin
- 1 teaspoon ground coriander
- 1 teaspoon turmeric powder
- 1/2 teaspoon chili powder (adjust to taste)
- 1 can (15 oz) chickpeas, drained and rinsed
- 1 can (14 oz) diced tomatoes
- 2 cups fresh spinach leaves
- Salt and pepper to taste
- Fresh cilantro for garnish (optional)
- Cooked brown rice for serving

Directions:

1. Heat olive oil in a large skillet over medium heat. Add the chopped onion and cook until softened, about 5 minutes.
2. Add minced garlic and grated ginger to the skillet. Cook for another 1-2 minutes until fragrant.
3. Stir in the ground cumin, ground coriander, turmeric powder, and chili powder. Cook for 1 minute, stirring constantly.
4. Add the drained chickpeas and diced tomatoes to the skillet. Stir to combine.

5. Reduce heat to low and simmer for 15-20 minutes, stirring occasionally, until the sauce thickens.
6. Stir in the fresh spinach leaves and cook until wilted, about 2-3 minutes.
7. Season with salt and pepper to taste.
8. Garnish with fresh cilantro if desired.
9. Serve hot over cooked brown rice.

Nutritional Information (per serving):
- Calories: 280
- Protein: 9g
- Fat: 8g
- Carbohydrates: 45g
- Fiber: 10g

Brown Rice and Edamame Salad

Total Time: 20 minutes
Number of Servings: 4

Ingredients:
- 1 cup brown rice, cooked
- 1 cup shelled edamame, cooked
- 1 red bell pepper, diced
- 1/2 cucumber, diced
- 1/4 cup chopped cilantro
- 2 tablespoons rice vinegar
- 1 tablespoon soy sauce
- 1 tablespoon sesame oil
- 1 teaspoon honey or maple syrup
- Salt and pepper to taste
- Sesame seeds for garnish (optional)

Directions:
1. In a large mixing bowl, combine the cooked brown rice, cooked edamame, diced red bell pepper, diced cucumber, and chopped cilantro.
2. In a small bowl, whisk together the rice vinegar, soy sauce, sesame oil, honey/maple syrup, salt, and pepper to make the dressing.
3. Pour the dressing over the salad ingredients and toss until well combined.
4. Sprinkle with sesame seeds for garnish if desired.
5. Serve immediately or refrigerate until ready to serve.

Nutritional Information (per serving):
- Calories: 250
- Protein: 10g

- Fat: 6g
- Carbohydrates: 40g
- Fiber: 6g

Whole Wheat Pita with Hummus and Veggies

Total Time: 10 minutes
Number of Servings: 2

Ingredients:
- 2 whole wheat pita bread rounds
- 1/2 cup hummus
- 1/2 cup mixed vegetables (carrots, cucumbers, bell peppers, etc.), thinly sliced or chopped
- Salt and pepper to taste

Directions:
1. Warm the whole wheat pita bread rounds in a toaster or oven if desired.
2. Spread each pita bread round with hummus.
3. Layer the mixed vegetables on top of the hummus.
4. Season with salt and pepper to taste.
5. Serve immediately.

Nutritional Information (per serving):
- Calories: 280
- Protein: 10g
- Fat: 10g
- Carbohydrates: 38g
- Fiber: 8g

Tofu and Vegetable Stir-Fry

Total Time: 25 minutes
Number of Servings: 4

Ingredients:
- 1 block (14 oz) extra-firm tofu, drained and pressed
- 2 tablespoons soy sauce
- 1 tablespoon sesame oil
- 1 tablespoon rice vinegar
- 1 tablespoon honey or maple syrup
- 2 cloves garlic, minced
- 1 teaspoon grated ginger

- 1 tablespoon vegetable oil
- 2 cups mixed vegetables (broccoli, bell peppers, snap peas, carrots, etc.), chopped
- Cooked brown rice for serving
- Sesame seeds for garnish (optional)
- Sliced green onions for garnish (optional)

Directions:
1. Cut the pressed tofu into cubes and place in a bowl.
2. In a separate bowl, whisk together the soy sauce, sesame oil, rice vinegar, honey/maple syrup, minced garlic, and grated ginger to make the sauce.
3. Pour the sauce over the tofu cubes and toss to coat. Let marinate for 10-15 minutes.
4. Heat vegetable oil in a large skillet or wok over medium-high heat.
5. Add the marinated tofu cubes to the skillet and cook until golden brown on all sides, about 5-7 minutes.
6. Remove the tofu from the skillet and set aside.
7. In the same skillet, add the chopped mixed vegetables and stir-fry for 3-5 minutes until crisp-tender.
8. Return the cooked tofu to the skillet and toss with the vegetables until heated through.
9. Serve the tofu and vegetable stir-fry over cooked brown rice.
10. Garnish with sesame seeds and sliced green onions if desired.

Nutritional Information (per serving):
- Calories: 280
- Protein: 14g
- Fat: 12g
- Carbohydrates: 32g
- Fiber: 6g

Roasted Beet and Arugula Salad with Walnuts

Total Time: 40 minutes
Number of Servings: 2

Ingredients:
- 2 medium beets, peeled and diced
- 2 cups arugula
- 1/4 cup crumbled feta cheese
- 1/4 cup chopped walnuts, toasted
- 2 tablespoons balsamic vinegar
- 1 tablespoon olive oil
- 1 teaspoon honey or maple syrup
- Salt and pepper to taste

Directions:

1. Preheat the oven to 400°F (200°C).
2. Place the diced beets on a baking sheet lined with parchment paper. Drizzle with olive oil and season with salt and pepper. Toss to coat.
3. Roast the beets in the preheated oven for 25-30 minutes until tender.
4. In a small bowl, whisk together the balsamic vinegar, olive oil, honey/maple syrup, salt, and pepper to make the dressing.
5. In a large mixing bowl, combine the roasted beets, arugula, crumbled feta cheese, and chopped walnuts.
6. Drizzle the dressing over the salad and toss until well combined.
7. Divide the salad into serving bowls and serve immediately.

Nutritional Information (per serving):

- Calories: 250
- Protein: 8g
- Fat: 16g
- Carbohydrates: 22g
- Fiber: 6g

Tuna and Avocado Salad on Whole Grain Crackers

Total Time: 10 minutes
Number of Servings: 2

Ingredients:

- 1 can (5 oz) tuna, drained
- 1 ripe avocado, mashed
- 1 tablespoon Greek yogurt
- 1 tablespoon lemon juice
- Salt and pepper to taste
- Whole grain crackers for serving

Directions:

1. In a bowl, combine the drained tuna, mashed avocado, Greek yogurt, lemon juice, salt, and pepper. Mix well until combined.
2. Spread the tuna and avocado mixture on whole grain crackers.
3. Serve immediately.

Nutritional Information (per serving):

- Calories: 250
- Protein: 20g
- Fat: 14g
- Carbohydrates: 15g
- Fiber: 7g

Mediterranean Quinoa Salad with Olives and Feta

Total Time: 25 minutes
Number of Servings: 4

Ingredients:
- 1 cup quinoa
- 2 cups water or vegetable broth
- 1 cup cherry tomatoes, halved
- 1/2 cup Kalamata olives, pitted and sliced
- 1/2 cup cucumber, diced
- 1/4 cup red onion, thinly sliced
- 1/4 cup crumbled feta cheese
- 2 tablespoons chopped fresh parsley
- 2 tablespoons extra virgin olive oil
- 1 tablespoon red wine vinegar
- Salt and pepper to taste

Directions:
1. Rinse the quinoa under cold water. In a saucepan, bring the water or vegetable broth to a boil. Add the quinoa, reduce heat to low, cover, and simmer for 15 minutes. Remove from heat and let sit for 5 minutes. Fluff with a fork.
2. In a large mixing bowl, combine the cooked quinoa, cherry tomatoes, Kalamata olives, cucumber, red onion, crumbled feta cheese, and chopped fresh parsley.
3. In a small bowl, whisk together the extra virgin olive oil, red wine vinegar, salt, and pepper to make the dressing.
4. Pour the dressing over the salad ingredients and toss until well combined.
5. Serve immediately or refrigerate until ready to serve.

Nutritional Information (per serving):
- Calories: 280
- Protein: 8g
- Fat: 14g
- Carbohydrates: 32g
- Fiber: 5g

Lentil and Sweet Potato Stew

Total Time: 40 minutes
Number of Servings: 6

Ingredients:
- 1 cup dried green lentils, rinsed and drained
- 2 sweet potatoes, peeled and diced
- 1 onion, diced
- 2 cloves garlic, minced
- 1 teaspoon ground cumin
- 1 teaspoon ground coriander
- 1/2 teaspoon smoked paprika
- 6 cups vegetable broth
- 1 can (14 oz) diced tomatoes
- 2 cups chopped kale or spinach
- Salt and pepper to taste
- Fresh parsley for garnish (optional)

Directions:
1. In a large pot, combine the dried green lentils, diced sweet potatoes, diced onion, minced garlic, ground cumin, ground coriander, smoked paprika, vegetable broth, and diced tomatoes.
2. Bring the mixture to a boil, then reduce heat to low and simmer for 25-30 minutes, until lentils and sweet potatoes are tender.
3. Stir in the chopped kale or spinach and cook for an additional 5 minutes until wilted.
4. Season with salt and pepper to taste.
5. Garnish with fresh parsley if desired.
6. Serve hot.

Nutritional Information (per serving):
- Calories: 280
- Protein: 14g
- Fat: 2g
- Carbohydrates: 50g
- Fiber: 15g

Black Bean and Corn Salad with Lime Dressing

Total Time: 15 minutes
Number of Servings: 4

Ingredients:
- 1 can (15 oz) black beans, drained and rinsed
- 1 cup frozen corn, thawed
- 1/2 red bell pepper, diced
- 1/4 cup red onion, finely chopped
- 1/4 cup chopped fresh cilantro
- Juice of 1 lime
- 2 tablespoons extra virgin olive oil
- 1 teaspoon ground cumin
- Salt and pepper to taste
- Optional: diced avocado for serving

Directions:
1. In a large mixing bowl, combine the black beans, corn, diced red bell pepper, chopped red onion, and chopped fresh cilantro.
2. In a small bowl, whisk together the lime juice, extra virgin olive oil, ground cumin, salt, and pepper to make the dressing.
3. Pour the dressing over the salad ingredients and toss until well combined.
4. Serve immediately, topped with diced avocado if desired.

Nutritional Information (per serving):
- Calories: 220
- Protein: 8g
- Fat: 8g
- Carbohydrates: 30g
- Fiber: 8g

Baked Falafel with Tzatziki Sauce

Total Time: 40 minutes
Number of Servings: 4

Ingredients:
- 1 can (15 oz) chickpeas, drained and rinsed
- 1/4 cup chopped fresh parsley
- 2 cloves garlic, minced
- 1 teaspoon ground cumin
- 1 teaspoon ground coriander

- 1/2 teaspoon paprika
- 1/4 teaspoon cayenne pepper
- Salt and pepper to taste
- 2 tablespoons olive oil
- Tzatziki sauce for serving

Directions:

1. Preheat the oven to 375°F (190°C). Line a baking sheet with parchment paper.
2. In a food processor, combine the chickpeas, chopped fresh parsley, minced garlic, ground cumin, ground coriander, paprika, cayenne pepper, salt, and pepper. Pulse until the mixture is well combined but still slightly chunky.
3. Form the mixture into small balls or patties and place them on the prepared baking sheet.
4. Drizzle the falafel with olive oil.
5. Bake in the preheated oven for 25-30 minutes, until golden brown and crispy.
6. Serve hot with tzatziki sauce.

Nutritional Information (per serving, excluding tzatziki sauce):

- Calories: 200
- Protein: 8g
- Fat: 8g
- Carbohydrates: 26g
- Fiber: 8g

Vegetable and Chickpea Buddha Bowl

Total Time: 30 minutes
Number of Servings: 2

Ingredients:

- 1 cup cooked quinoa or brown rice
- 1 cup cooked chickpeas
- 2 cups mixed vegetables (such as broccoli, bell peppers, carrots, zucchini), chopped
- 2 tablespoons olive oil
- 1 teaspoon ground cumin
- 1 teaspoon smoked paprika
- Salt and pepper to taste
- Hummus for serving
- Lemon wedges for serving

Directions:

1. In a large skillet, heat olive oil over medium heat. Add the mixed vegetables and sauté until tender, about 5-7 minutes.

2. Season the vegetables with ground cumin, smoked paprika, salt, and pepper. Stir to coat evenly.
3. Divide the cooked quinoa or brown rice between serving bowls.
4. Top with cooked chickpeas and sautéed vegetables.
5. Serve with a dollop of hummus and lemon wedges on the side.

Nutritional Information (per serving):

- Calories: 400
- Protein: 15g
- Fat: 14g
- Carbohydrates: 55g
- Fiber: 12g

Dinner

Baked Salmon with Asparagus and Quinoa

Total Time: 30 minutes
Number of Servings: 4

Ingredients:
- 4 salmon fillets
- 1 bunch asparagus, trimmed
- 1 cup quinoa
- 2 cups water or vegetable broth
- 2 tablespoons olive oil
- 2 cloves garlic, minced
- 1 teaspoon lemon zest
- 1 tablespoon lemon juice
- Salt and pepper to taste
- Fresh parsley for garnish (optional)

Directions:
1. Preheat the oven to 400°F (200°C). Line a baking sheet with parchment paper.
2. Place the salmon fillets on one side of the baking sheet and the trimmed asparagus on the other side.
3. Drizzle olive oil over the salmon and asparagus. Sprinkle minced garlic, lemon zest, and lemon juice over the top. Season with salt and pepper.
4. Bake in the preheated oven for 15-20 minutes until the salmon is cooked through and the asparagus is tender.
5. While the salmon and asparagus are baking, rinse the quinoa under cold water. In a saucepan, bring the water or vegetable broth to a boil. Add the quinoa, reduce heat to low, cover, and simmer for 15 minutes. Remove from heat and let sit for 5 minutes. Fluff with a fork.
6. Serve the baked salmon and asparagus over cooked quinoa.
7. Garnish with fresh parsley if desired.
8. Serve hot.

Nutritional Information (per serving):
- Calories: 400
- Protein: 30g
- Fat: 18g
- Carbohydrates: 30g
- Fiber: 5g

Grilled Chicken with Roasted Vegetables

Total Time: 40 minutes
Number of Servings: 4

Ingredients:
- 4 boneless, skinless chicken breasts
- 2 bell peppers, sliced
- 1 zucchini, sliced
- 1 red onion, sliced
- 2 tablespoons olive oil
- 2 cloves garlic, minced
- 1 teaspoon Italian seasoning
- Salt and pepper to taste
- Fresh basil for garnish (optional)

Directions:
1. Preheat the grill to medium-high heat.
2. In a large bowl, toss the sliced bell peppers, zucchini, and red onion with olive oil, minced garlic, Italian seasoning, salt, and pepper.
3. Place the chicken breasts and seasoned vegetables on the grill.
4. Grill the chicken for 6-8 minutes per side, or until cooked through and no longer pink in the center.
5. Grill the vegetables for 5-7 minutes, or until tender and lightly charred.
6. Remove the chicken and vegetables from the grill.
7. Serve the grilled chicken with roasted vegetables.
8. Garnish with fresh basil if desired.
9. Serve hot.

Nutritional Information (per serving):
- Calories: 300
- Protein: 35g
- Fat: 12g
- Carbohydrates: 15g
- Fiber: 5g

Lentil and Spinach Stuffed Peppers

Total Time: 50 minutes
Number of Servings: 4

Ingredients:
- 4 large bell peppers, any color
- 1 cup cooked lentils

- 2 cups fresh spinach, chopped
- 1 cup cooked brown rice
- 1/2 cup diced tomatoes
- 1/4 cup chopped red onion
- 2 cloves garlic, minced
- 1 teaspoon dried oregano
- 1/2 teaspoon smoked paprika
- Salt and pepper to taste
- 1/4 cup shredded mozzarella cheese (optional)

Directions:
1. Preheat the oven to 375°F (190°C). Slice the tops off the bell peppers and remove the seeds and membranes.
2. In a large mixing bowl, combine the cooked lentils, chopped spinach, cooked brown rice, diced tomatoes, chopped red onion, minced garlic, dried oregano, smoked paprika, salt, and pepper.
3. Stuff the mixture into the hollowed-out bell peppers.
4. Place the stuffed peppers in a baking dish. If using shredded mozzarella cheese, sprinkle it on top of the stuffed peppers.
5. Cover the baking dish with foil and bake in the preheated oven for 30-35 minutes, or until the peppers are tender.
6. Remove the foil and bake for an additional 5 minutes to melt the cheese (if using).
7. Serve hot.

Nutritional Information (per serving):
- Calories: 250
- Protein: 15g
- Fat: 3g
- Carbohydrates: 45g
- Fiber: 10g

Quinoa and Black Bean Tacos with Avocado

Total Time: 25 minutes
Number of Servings: 4 (2 tacos per serving)

Ingredients:
- 1 cup quinoa
- 2 cups water or vegetable broth
- 1 can (15 oz) black beans, drained and rinsed
- 1 teaspoon ground cumin
- 1 teaspoon chili powder
- Salt and pepper to taste
- 8 corn tortillas

- 1 ripe avocado, sliced
- Fresh cilantro for garnish (optional)
- Lime wedges for serving

Directions:
1. Rinse the quinoa under cold water. In a saucepan, bring the water or vegetable broth to a boil. Add the quinoa, reduce heat to low, cover, and simmer for 15 minutes. Remove from heat and let sit for 5 minutes. Fluff with a fork.
2. In a separate saucepan, heat the black beans over medium heat. Stir in the ground cumin, chili powder, salt, and pepper. Cook for 5-7 minutes until heated through.
3. Warm the corn tortillas in a dry skillet over medium heat, about 1 minute per side.
4. Assemble the tacos by filling each tortilla with cooked quinoa, black beans, and sliced avocado.
5. Garnish with fresh cilantro if desired and serve with lime wedges on the side.

Nutritional Information (per serving, 2 tacos):
- Calories: 400
- Protein: 15g
- Fat: 10g
- Carbohydrates: 65g
- Fiber: 12g

Turkey Meatballs with Whole Grain Spaghetti

Total Time: 45 minutes
Number of Servings: 4

Ingredients:
- 1 lb ground turkey
- 1/4 cup breadcrumbs (whole wheat if available)
- 1/4 cup grated Parmesan cheese
- 1 egg
- 2 cloves garlic, minced
- 2 tablespoons chopped fresh parsley
- 1 teaspoon dried oregano
- Salt and pepper to taste
- 8 oz whole grain spaghetti
- 2 cups marinara sauce
- Fresh basil for garnish (optional)

Directions:
1. Preheat the oven to 400°F (200°C). Line a baking sheet with parchment paper.

2. In a large mixing bowl, combine the ground turkey, breadcrumbs, grated Parmesan cheese, egg, minced garlic, chopped fresh parsley, dried oregano, salt, and pepper. Mix until well combined.
3. Roll the mixture into small meatballs and place them on the prepared baking sheet.
4. Bake in the preheated oven for 20-25 minutes, or until the meatballs are cooked through and lightly browned.
5. While the meatballs are baking, cook the whole grain spaghetti according to package instructions. Drain and set aside.
6. Heat the marinara sauce in a saucepan over medium heat.
7. Serve the turkey meatballs over cooked whole grain spaghetti, topped with marinara sauce.
8. Garnish with fresh basil if desired.
9. Serve hot.

Nutritional Information (per serving):
- Calories: 400
- Protein: 25g
- Fat: 10g
- Carbohydrates: 45g
- Fiber: 8g

Vegetable Stir-Fry with Brown Rice

Total Time: 25 minutes
Number of Servings: 4

Ingredients:
- 2 cups cooked brown rice
- 1 tablespoon sesame oil
- 2 cloves garlic, minced
- 1 tablespoon grated ginger
- 2 cups mixed vegetables (bell peppers, broccoli, snap peas, carrots, etc.), sliced
- 1 cup tofu, diced (optional)
- 3 tablespoons soy sauce
- 1 tablespoon rice vinegar
- 1 teaspoon honey or maple syrup
- Salt and pepper to taste
- Sesame seeds for garnish (optional)
- Sliced green onions for garnish (optional)

Directions:
1. Heat sesame oil in a large skillet or wok over medium-high heat.
2. Add minced garlic and grated ginger, sauté for 1 minute until fragrant.

3. Add mixed vegetables (and tofu if using) to the skillet. Stir-fry for 3-5 minutes until vegetables are tender-crisp.
4. In a small bowl, whisk together soy sauce, rice vinegar, honey/maple syrup, salt, and pepper.
5. Pour the sauce over the vegetables in the skillet. Stir well to coat evenly.
6. Serve the vegetable stir-fry over cooked brown rice.
7. Garnish with sesame seeds and sliced green onions if desired.
8. Serve hot.

Nutritional Information (per serving):
- Calories: 300
- Protein: 10g
- Fat: 8g
- Carbohydrates: 50g
- Fiber: 8g

Baked Cod with Sweet Potato Mash

Total Time: 30 minutes
Number of Servings: 4

Ingredients:
- 4 cod fillets
- 2 large sweet potatoes, peeled and diced
- 2 tablespoons olive oil
- 2 cloves garlic, minced
- 1 teaspoon smoked paprika
- Salt and pepper to taste
- Fresh parsley for garnish (optional)

Directions:
1. Preheat the oven to 400°F (200°C). Line a baking sheet with parchment paper.
2. Place the diced sweet potatoes on the prepared baking sheet. Drizzle with olive oil and sprinkle minced garlic, smoked paprika, salt, and pepper over the top. Toss to coat evenly.
3. Roast the sweet potatoes in the preheated oven for 20-25 minutes, until tender and lightly browned.
4. Place the cod fillets on a separate baking sheet lined with parchment paper. Drizzle with olive oil and season with salt and pepper.
5. Bake the cod fillets in the preheated oven for 12-15 minutes, or until the fish flakes easily with a fork.
6. Serve the baked cod with roasted sweet potato mash.
7. Garnish with fresh parsley if desired.
8. Serve hot.

Nutritional Information (per serving):
- Calories: 250
- Protein: 25g
- Fat: 8g
- Carbohydrates: 20g
- Fiber: 4g

Chickpea and Cauliflower Curry with Brown Rice

Total Time: 40 minutes
Number of Servings: 4

Ingredients:
- 1 cup brown rice
- 2 cups water or vegetable broth
- 1 tablespoon coconut oil
- 1 onion, diced
- 3 cloves garlic, minced
- 1 tablespoon grated ginger
- 1 tablespoon curry powder
- 1 teaspoon ground cumin
- 1 teaspoon ground coriander
- 1/2 teaspoon turmeric
- 1 can (15 oz) chickpeas, drained and rinsed
- 1 head cauliflower, cut into florets
- 1 can (14 oz) diced tomatoes
- 1 cup coconut milk
- Salt and pepper to taste
- Fresh cilantro for garnish (optional)

Directions:
1. Rinse the brown rice under cold water. In a saucepan, bring the water or vegetable broth to a boil. Add the brown rice, reduce heat to low, cover, and simmer for 30 minutes. Remove from heat and let sit for 5 minutes. Fluff with a fork.
2. In a large skillet or pot, heat coconut oil over medium heat. Add diced onion, minced garlic, and grated ginger. Sauté for 2-3 minutes until softened and fragrant.
3. Add curry powder, ground cumin, ground coriander, and turmeric to the skillet. Cook for 1 minute, stirring constantly.
4. Add chickpeas, cauliflower florets, diced tomatoes (with juices), and coconut milk to the skillet. Stir to combine.
5. Cover and simmer for 15-20 minutes, until the cauliflower is tender.
6. Season with salt and pepper to taste.
7. Serve the chickpea and cauliflower curry over cooked brown rice.

8. Garnish with fresh cilantro if desired.
9. Serve hot.

Nutritional Information (per serving):
- Calories: 350
- Protein: 12g
- Fat: 15g
- Carbohydrates: 45g
- Fiber: 10g

Grilled Tofu with Quinoa and Steamed Broccoli

Total Time: 30 minutes
Number of Servings: 4

Ingredients:
- 1 cup quinoa
- 2 cups water or vegetable broth
- 1 block (14 oz) firm tofu, drained and pressed
- 2 tablespoons soy sauce
- 1 tablespoon sesame oil
- 1 tablespoon maple syrup
- 1 teaspoon grated ginger
- 1 clove garlic, minced
- 4 cups broccoli florets
- Salt and pepper to taste
- Lemon wedges for serving

Directions:
1. Rinse the quinoa under cold water. In a saucepan, bring the water or vegetable broth to a boil. Add the quinoa, reduce heat to low, cover, and simmer for 15 minutes. Remove from heat and let sit for 5 minutes. Fluff with a fork.
2. Cut the pressed tofu into cubes and place in a bowl. In a separate bowl, whisk together soy sauce, sesame oil, maple syrup, grated ginger, and minced garlic. Pour over the tofu cubes and let marinate for 10-15 minutes.
3. Preheat the grill or grill pan over medium-high heat. Grill the tofu cubes for 3-4 minutes per side, until lightly charred.
4. Steam the broccoli florets until tender, about 5 minutes.
5. Serve grilled tofu over cooked quinoa with steamed broccoli on the side.
6. Season with salt and pepper to taste.
7. Serve with lemon wedges for squeezing over the tofu and broccoli.
8. Serve hot.

Nutritional Information (per serving):
- Calories: 350
- Protein: 20g
- Fat: 12g
- Carbohydrates: 40g
- Fiber: 8g

Mediterranean Baked Chicken with Olives and Tomatoes

Total Time: 45 minutes
Number of Servings: 4

Ingredients:
- 4 boneless, skinless chicken breasts
- 1 cup cherry tomatoes, halved
- 1/2 cup Kalamata olives, pitted
- 2 cloves garlic, minced
- 2 tablespoons extra virgin olive oil
- 1 tablespoon balsamic vinegar
- 1 teaspoon dried oregano
- 1 teaspoon dried basil
- Salt and pepper to taste
- Fresh parsley for garnish (optional)

Directions:
1. Preheat the oven to 375°F (190°C). Line a baking dish with parchment paper.
2. Place the chicken breasts in the prepared baking dish. Arrange cherry tomatoes and Kalamata olives around the chicken.
3. In a small bowl, whisk together minced garlic, extra virgin olive oil, balsamic vinegar, dried oregano, dried basil, salt, and pepper.
4. Pour the olive oil mixture over the chicken, tomatoes, and olives.
5. Bake in the preheated oven for 25-30 minutes, or until the chicken is cooked through and no longer pink in the center.
6. Garnish with fresh parsley if desired.
7. Serve hot.

Nutritional Information (per serving):
- Calories: 300
- Protein: 30g
- Fat: 12g
- Carbohydrates: 10g
- Fiber: 2g

Lentil Shepherd's Pie with Sweet Potato Topping

Total Time: 1 hour
Number of Servings: 6

Ingredients:
- 2 large sweet potatoes, peeled and cubed
- 1 cup green lentils, rinsed
- 2 cups vegetable broth
- 1 onion, diced
- 2 carrots, diced
- 2 celery stalks, diced
- 2 cloves garlic, minced
- 1 cup frozen peas
- 2 tablespoons tomato paste
- 1 tablespoon Worcestershire sauce (vegan if preferred)
- 1 teaspoon dried thyme
- Salt and pepper to taste
- 2 tablespoons olive oil
- Fresh parsley for garnish (optional)

Directions:
1. Preheat the oven to 375°F (190°C).
2. Place the sweet potato cubes in a pot of water. Bring to a boil and cook until tender, about 15-20 minutes. Drain and mash with a fork or potato masher. Set aside.
3. In a separate pot, combine the green lentils and vegetable broth. Bring to a boil, then reduce heat and simmer for 20-25 minutes until lentils are tender and most of the liquid is absorbed.
4. In a large skillet, heat olive oil over medium heat. Add diced onion, carrots, celery, and minced garlic. Sauté for 5-7 minutes until vegetables are softened.
5. Stir in cooked green lentils, frozen peas, tomato paste, Worcestershire sauce, dried thyme, salt, and pepper. Cook for an additional 5 minutes, stirring occasionally.
6. Transfer the lentil and vegetable mixture to a baking dish. Spread the mashed sweet potatoes evenly over the top.
7. Bake in the preheated oven for 20-25 minutes until the sweet potato topping is lightly browned.
8. Garnish with fresh parsley if desired.
9. Serve hot.

Nutritional Information (per serving):
- Calories: 300
- Protein: 10g
- Fat: 5g
- Carbohydrates: 50g
- Fiber: 10g

Grilled Shrimp Skewers with Quinoa Salad

Total Time: 30 minutes
Number of Servings: 4

Ingredients:
- 1 lb large shrimp, peeled and deveined
- 1 lemon, juiced and zested
- 2 tablespoons olive oil
- 2 cloves garlic, minced
- 1 teaspoon smoked paprika
- Salt and pepper to taste
- 1 cup quinoa
- 2 cups water or vegetable broth
- 1 cucumber, diced
- 1 cup cherry tomatoes, halved
- 1/4 cup chopped fresh parsley
- 1/4 cup crumbled feta cheese (optional)

Directions:
1. In a large bowl, combine shrimp, lemon juice and zest, olive oil, minced garlic, smoked paprika, salt, and pepper. Toss to coat shrimp evenly. Let marinate for 15-20 minutes.
2. Preheat the grill to medium-high heat. Thread marinated shrimp onto skewers.
3. Grill shrimp skewers for 2-3 minutes per side until shrimp are pink and opaque.
4. Rinse quinoa under cold water. In a saucepan, bring water or vegetable broth to a boil. Add quinoa, reduce heat to low, cover, and simmer for 15 minutes. Remove from heat and let sit for 5 minutes. Fluff with a fork.
5. In a large mixing bowl, combine cooked quinoa, diced cucumber, halved cherry tomatoes, chopped fresh parsley, and crumbled feta cheese (if using).
6. Serve grilled shrimp skewers with quinoa salad.
7. Serve hot or at room temperature.

Nutritional Information (per serving):
- Calories: 350
- Protein: 25g
- Fat: 10g
- Carbohydrates: 40g
- Fiber: 6g

Turkey and Vegetable Stir-Fry

Total Time: 25 minutes
Number of Servings: 4

Ingredients:
- 1 lb ground turkey
- 2 tablespoons soy sauce
- 1 tablespoon sesame oil
- 1 tablespoon cornstarch
- 2 tablespoons olive oil
- 1 onion, thinly sliced
- 2 bell peppers, thinly sliced
- 1 cup broccoli florets
- 1 cup snap peas
- 2 cloves garlic, minced
- 1 teaspoon grated ginger
- Salt and pepper to taste
- Cooked brown rice for serving

Directions:
1. In a small bowl, combine ground turkey, soy sauce, sesame oil, and cornstarch. Mix well and set aside.
2. Heat olive oil in a large skillet or wok over medium-high heat. Add sliced onion and bell peppers. Stir-fry for 3-4 minutes until vegetables are slightly softened.
3. Add broccoli florets, snap peas, minced garlic, and grated ginger to the skillet. Stir-fry for an additional 2-3 minutes.
4. Push vegetables to one side of the skillet and add the ground turkey mixture to the empty side. Cook, breaking up the turkey with a spoon, until no longer pink, about 5-7 minutes.
5. Stir the cooked turkey into the vegetables. Season with salt and pepper to taste.
6. Serve turkey and vegetable stir-fry over cooked brown rice.
7. Serve hot.

Nutritional Information (per serving):
- Calories: 300
- Protein: 25g
- Fat: 12g
- Carbohydrates: 20g
- Fiber: 5g

Stuffed Eggplant with Quinoa and Vegetables

Total Time: 50 minutes
Number of Servings: 4

Ingredients:
- 2 large eggplants
- 1 cup quinoa
- 2 cups water or vegetable broth
- 1 onion, diced
- 2 cloves garlic, minced
- 1 bell pepper, diced
- 1 zucchini, diced
- 1 cup cherry tomatoes, halved
- 1/4 cup chopped fresh parsley
- 1/4 cup crumbled feta cheese (optional)
- 2 tablespoons olive oil
- Salt and pepper to taste

Directions:
1. Preheat the oven to 375°F (190°C).
2. Cut each eggplant in half lengthwise. Scoop out the flesh, leaving about a 1/4-inch thick shell. Chop the eggplant flesh and set aside.
3. Rinse quinoa under cold water. In a saucepan, bring water or vegetable broth to a boil. Add quinoa, reduce heat to low, cover, and simmer for 15 minutes. Remove from heat and let sit for 5 minutes. Fluff with a fork.
4. In a large skillet, heat olive oil over medium heat. Add diced onion and minced garlic. Sauté for 2-3 minutes until softened.
5. Add chopped eggplant flesh, diced bell pepper, and diced zucchini to the skillet. Cook for 5-7 minutes until vegetables are tender.
6. Stir in cooked quinoa, halved cherry tomatoes, chopped fresh parsley, and crumbled feta cheese (if using). Season with salt and pepper to taste.
7. Stuff the eggplant shells with the quinoa and vegetable mixture.
8. Place stuffed eggplants on a baking sheet. Bake in the preheated oven for 20-25 minutes until eggplants are tender.
9. Serve hot.

Nutritional Information (per serving):
- Calories: 300
- Protein: 10g
- Fat: 10g
- Carbohydrates: 40g
- Fiber: 10g

Roasted Chicken with Brussels Sprouts and Wild Rice

Total Time: 1 hour
Number of Servings: 4

Ingredients:
- 4 bone-in, skin-on chicken thighs
- 2 cups Brussels sprouts, halved
- 1 cup wild rice
- 2 cups chicken broth
- 2 tablespoons olive oil
- 2 cloves garlic, minced
- 1 teaspoon dried thyme
- Salt and pepper to taste
- Lemon wedges for serving

Directions:
1. Preheat the oven to 400°F (200°C). Line a baking sheet with parchment paper.
2. In a saucepan, combine wild rice and chicken broth. Bring to a boil, then reduce heat to low, cover, and simmer for 40-45 minutes until rice is tender and liquid is absorbed.
3. Place chicken thighs on one side of the prepared baking sheet. Arrange halved Brussels sprouts on the other side.
4. Drizzle olive oil over chicken thighs and Brussels sprouts. Sprinkle minced garlic and dried thyme evenly over the top. Season with salt and pepper.
5. Roast in the preheated oven for 30-35 minutes until chicken is cooked through and Brussels sprouts are tender and lightly browned.
6. Serve roasted chicken with Brussels sprouts and wild rice.
7. Serve with lemon wedges for squeezing over the chicken and vegetables.
8. Serve hot.

Nutritional Information (per serving):
- Calories: 400
- Protein: 25g
- Fat: 18g
- Carbohydrates: 30g
- Fiber: 5g

Poultry and Meat

Lemon Herb Grilled Chicken Breast

Total Time: 30 minutes
Number of Servings: 4

Ingredients:
- 4 boneless, skinless chicken breasts
- Zest and juice of 1 lemon
- 2 tablespoons olive oil
- 2 cloves garlic, minced
- 1 teaspoon dried thyme
- 1 teaspoon dried rosemary
- Salt and pepper to taste
- Fresh parsley for garnish (optional)

Directions:
1. In a small bowl, whisk together lemon zest, lemon juice, olive oil, minced garlic, dried thyme, dried rosemary, salt, and pepper.
2. Place chicken breasts in a shallow dish or resealable plastic bag. Pour the marinade over the chicken, ensuring it's evenly coated. Marinate in the refrigerator for at least 30 minutes, or up to 4 hours.
3. Preheat the grill to medium-high heat. Remove chicken from marinade and discard excess marinade.
4. Grill chicken breasts for 6-8 minutes per side, or until cooked through and no longer pink in the center.
5. Garnish with fresh parsley if desired.
6. Serve hot.

Nutritional Information (per serving):
- Calories: 250
- Protein: 30g
- Fat: 12g
- Carbohydrates: 2g
- Fiber: 0g

Turkey Chili with Black Beans

Total Time: 1 hour
Number of Servings: 6

Ingredients:
- 1 lb ground turkey
- 1 onion, diced
- 2 cloves garlic, minced
- 1 bell pepper, diced
- 1 can (15 oz) black beans, drained and rinsed
- 1 can (14 oz) diced tomatoes
- 2 cups chicken broth
- 2 tablespoons chili powder
- 1 teaspoon ground cumin
- 1 teaspoon paprika
- Salt and pepper to taste
- Chopped fresh cilantro for garnish (optional)
- Greek yogurt for topping (optional)
- Shredded cheddar cheese for topping (optional)

Directions:
1. In a large pot or Dutch oven, cook ground turkey over medium heat until browned, breaking it up with a spoon as it cooks.
2. Add diced onion and minced garlic to the pot. Sauté for 2-3 minutes until softened.
3. Stir in diced bell pepper, black beans, diced tomatoes (with juices), chicken broth, chili powder, ground cumin, paprika, salt, and pepper.
4. Bring the chili to a simmer. Reduce heat to low, cover, and simmer for 30-40 minutes, stirring occasionally.
5. Taste and adjust seasoning if necessary.
6. Serve hot, garnished with chopped fresh cilantro, Greek yogurt, and shredded cheddar cheese if desired.

Nutritional Information (per serving):
- Calories: 300
- Protein: 25g
- Fat: 10g
- Carbohydrates: 20g
- Fiber: 6g

Baked Chicken Thighs with Rosemary and Garlic

Total Time: 40 minutes
Number of Servings: 4

Ingredients:
- 4 bone-in, skin-on chicken thighs
- 2 tablespoons olive oil
- 4 cloves garlic, minced
- 2 tablespoons chopped fresh rosemary
- Salt and pepper to taste
- Lemon wedges for serving

Directions:
1. Preheat the oven to 400°F (200°C). Line a baking sheet with parchment paper.
2. Pat chicken thighs dry with paper towels and place them on the prepared baking sheet.
3. In a small bowl, mix together olive oil, minced garlic, chopped fresh rosemary, salt, and pepper.
4. Rub the garlic rosemary mixture over the chicken thighs, ensuring they are evenly coated.
5. Bake in the preheated oven for 30-35 minutes, or until the chicken is cooked through and the skin is crispy and golden brown.
6. Serve hot with lemon wedges for squeezing over the chicken.

Nutritional Information (per serving):
- Calories: 350
- Protein: 25g
- Fat: 20g
- Carbohydrates: 0g
- Fiber: 0g

Turkey and Spinach Stuffed Peppers

Total Time: 1 hour
Number of Servings: 4

Ingredients:
- 4 large bell peppers, any color
- 1 lb ground turkey
- 1 onion, diced
- 2 cloves garlic, minced
- 2 cups fresh spinach, chopped
- 1 cup cooked quinoa

- 1 can (14 oz) diced tomatoes, drained
- 1 teaspoon Italian seasoning
- Salt and pepper to taste
- Shredded mozzarella cheese for topping (optional)
- Chopped fresh parsley for garnish (optional)

Directions:

1. Preheat the oven to 375°F (190°C). Slice the tops off the bell peppers and remove the seeds and membranes.
2. In a skillet, cook ground turkey over medium heat until browned. Add diced onion and minced garlic, and sauté until softened.
3. Stir in chopped spinach and cook until wilted.
4. Add cooked quinoa, diced tomatoes, Italian seasoning, salt, and pepper to the skillet. Stir to combine.
5. Stuff the bell peppers with the turkey and spinach mixture.
6. Place stuffed bell peppers in a baking dish. Cover with foil and bake in the preheated oven for 30 minutes.
7. Remove foil, sprinkle shredded mozzarella cheese over the top of each stuffed pepper if desired, and bake for an additional 10 minutes until cheese is melted and bubbly.
8. Garnish with chopped fresh parsley if desired.
9. Serve hot.

Nutritional Information (per serving):

- Calories: 300
- Protein: 25g
- Fat: 10g
- Carbohydrates: 20g
- Fiber: 4g

Chicken and Vegetable Kebabs

Total Time: 30 minutes
Number of Servings: 4

Ingredients:

- 1 lb boneless, skinless chicken breasts, cut into cubes
- 1 bell pepper, cut into chunks
- 1 zucchini, sliced
- 1 red onion, cut into chunks
- 8-10 cherry tomatoes
- 2 tablespoons olive oil
- 2 tablespoons balsamic vinegar
- 2 cloves garlic, minced

- 1 teaspoon dried oregano
- Salt and pepper to taste
- Wooden skewers, soaked in water for 30 minutes

Directions:
1. Preheat the grill to medium-high heat.
2. Thread chicken cubes, bell pepper chunks, zucchini slices, red onion chunks, and cherry tomatoes onto the soaked wooden skewers, alternating as desired.
3. In a small bowl, whisk together olive oil, balsamic vinegar, minced garlic, dried oregano, salt, and pepper.
4. Brush the marinade over the chicken and vegetable kebabs, ensuring they are evenly coated.
5. Grill the kebabs for 10-12 minutes, turning occasionally, until chicken is cooked through and vegetables are tender and lightly charred.
6. Serve hot.

Nutritional Information (per serving):
- Calories: 250
- Protein: 25g
- Fat: 10g
- Carbohydrates: 10g
- Fiber: 2g

Spicy Turkey Lettuce Wraps

Total Time: 30 minutes
Number of Servings: 4

Ingredients:
- 1 lb ground turkey
- 1 tablespoon olive oil
- 1 onion, diced
- 2 cloves garlic, minced
- 1 bell pepper, diced
- 1 tablespoon chili powder
- 1 teaspoon cumin
- 1/2 teaspoon paprika
- Salt and pepper to taste
- 1/4 cup chopped fresh cilantro
- 8 large lettuce leaves
- Optional toppings: diced tomatoes, avocado, Greek yogurt

Directions:

1. Heat olive oil in a large skillet over medium-high heat. Add diced onion, minced garlic, and diced bell pepper. Cook for 2-3 minutes until softened.
2. Add ground turkey to the skillet. Cook, breaking it up with a spoon, until browned and cooked through.
3. Stir in chili powder, cumin, paprika, salt, and pepper. Cook for an additional 2-3 minutes to allow the flavors to meld.
4. Remove from heat and stir in chopped fresh cilantro.
5. Spoon the turkey mixture onto lettuce leaves. Top with diced tomatoes, avocado, and Greek yogurt if desired.
6. Serve hot.

Nutritional Information (per serving):

- Calories: 250
- Protein: 25g
- Fat: 10g
- Carbohydrates: 10g
- Fiber: 2g

Baked Chicken with Tomato and Basil

Total Time: 40 minutes
Number of Servings: 4

Ingredients:

- 4 boneless, skinless chicken breasts
- 2 cups cherry tomatoes, halved
- 1/4 cup chopped fresh basil
- 2 cloves garlic, minced
- 2 tablespoons balsamic vinegar
- 2 tablespoons olive oil
- Salt and pepper to taste

Directions:

1. Preheat the oven to 400°F (200°C). Line a baking sheet with parchment paper.
2. Place chicken breasts on the prepared baking sheet.
3. In a bowl, combine cherry tomatoes, chopped fresh basil, minced garlic, balsamic vinegar, olive oil, salt, and pepper. Toss to coat tomatoes evenly.
4. Spoon the tomato mixture over the chicken breasts.
5. Bake in the preheated oven for 25-30 minutes, or until chicken is cooked through and tomatoes are softened and slightly caramelized.
6. Serve hot.

Nutritional Information (per serving):
- Calories: 300
- Protein: 30g
- Fat: 12g
- Carbohydrates: 10g
- Fiber: 2g

Turkey Meatloaf with Oats

Total Time: 1 hour
Number of Servings: 6

Ingredients:
- 1 lb ground turkey
- 1 cup rolled oats
- 1 onion, finely chopped
- 2 cloves garlic, minced
- 1 carrot, grated
- 1/4 cup ketchup
- 2 tablespoons Worcestershire sauce
- 1 teaspoon dried thyme
- 1 teaspoon dried oregano
- Salt and pepper to taste
- 1 egg, beaten
- 1/4 cup barbecue sauce

Directions:
1. Preheat the oven to 375°F (190°C). Grease a loaf pan with olive oil or non-stick cooking spray.
2. In a large bowl, combine ground turkey, rolled oats, chopped onion, minced garlic, grated carrot, ketchup, Worcestershire sauce, dried thyme, dried oregano, salt, pepper, and beaten egg. Mix until well combined.
3. Press the turkey mixture into the prepared loaf pan.
4. Spread barbecue sauce evenly over the top of the meatloaf.
5. Bake in the preheated oven for 45-50 minutes, or until cooked through and golden brown on top.
6. Let the meatloaf rest for 5 minutes before slicing.
7. Serve hot.

Nutritional Information (per serving):
- Calories: 250
- Protein: 20g
- Fat: 10g
- Carbohydrates: 15g
- Fiber: 2g

Chicken and Broccoli Stir-Fry

Total Time: 30 minutes
Number of Servings: 4

Ingredients:
- 1 lb boneless, skinless chicken breasts, cut into strips
- 2 tablespoons soy sauce
- 1 tablespoon sesame oil
- 2 cloves garlic, minced
- 1 teaspoon grated ginger
- 2 cups broccoli florets
- 1 bell pepper, sliced
- 1 carrot, sliced
- 1/4 cup chicken broth
- 1 tablespoon cornstarch
- Salt and pepper to taste
- Cooked brown rice for serving

Directions:
1. In a bowl, combine chicken strips with soy sauce, sesame oil, minced garlic, and grated ginger. Toss to coat chicken evenly. Let marinate for 15 minutes.
2. Heat a large skillet or wok over medium-high heat. Add marinated chicken strips and cook until browned and cooked through.
3. Add broccoli florets, sliced bell pepper, and sliced carrot to the skillet. Stir-fry for 3-4 minutes until vegetables are tender-crisp.
4. In a small bowl, whisk together chicken broth and cornstarch to make a slurry. Pour the slurry into the skillet and stir well.
5. Cook for an additional 1-2 minutes until the sauce has thickened.
6. Season with salt and pepper to taste.
7. Serve chicken and broccoli stir-fry over cooked brown rice.
8. Serve hot.

Nutritional Information (per serving):
- Calories: 300
- Protein: 25g
- Fat: 10g
- Carbohydrates: 20g
- Fiber: 4g

Grilled Turkey Burgers with Avocado

Total Time: 30 minutes
Number of Servings: 4

Ingredients:
- 1 lb ground turkey
- 1/4 cup breadcrumbs
- 1 egg
- 1/4 cup chopped fresh parsley
- 1 teaspoon garlic powder
- 1 teaspoon onion powder
- Salt and pepper to taste
- 1 avocado, sliced
- 4 whole wheat burger buns
- Optional toppings: lettuce, tomato, red onion, mustard, mayonnaise

Directions:
1. Preheat the grill to medium-high heat.
2. In a bowl, combine ground turkey, breadcrumbs, egg, chopped fresh parsley, garlic powder, onion powder, salt, and pepper. Mix until well combined.
3. Divide the turkey mixture into 4 equal portions and shape into burger patties.
4. Grill the turkey burgers for 5-6 minutes per side, or until cooked through and no longer pink in the center.
5. Toast the whole wheat burger buns on the grill for 1-2 minutes until lightly browned.
6. Assemble the burgers by placing a turkey patty on each bun, topping with sliced avocado, and adding any other desired toppings.
7. Serve hot.

Nutritional Information (per serving):
- Calories: 350
- Protein: 25g
- Fat: 15g
- Carbohydrates: 25g
- Fiber: 5g

Soup and Salad

Tomato Basil Soup

Total Time: 45 minutes
Number of Servings: 4

Ingredients:
- 2 tablespoons olive oil
- 1 onion, diced
- 2 cloves garlic, minced
- 4 cups fresh tomatoes, chopped (or 2 cans diced tomatoes)
- 1 tablespoon tomato paste
- 2 cups vegetable broth
- 1/4 cup chopped fresh basil
- Salt and pepper to taste
- Optional garnish: chopped fresh basil, croutons

Directions:
1. Heat olive oil in a large pot over medium heat. Add diced onion and minced garlic. Cook for 5-7 minutes until softened.
2. Add chopped tomatoes and tomato paste to the pot. Cook for an additional 5 minutes.
3. Pour in vegetable broth and bring the soup to a simmer. Cook for 20-25 minutes.
4. Stir in chopped fresh basil. Season with salt and pepper to taste.
5. Use an immersion blender to blend the soup until smooth. Alternatively, transfer the soup to a blender and blend until smooth, then return it to the pot.
6. Serve hot, garnished with additional chopped fresh basil and croutons if desired.

Nutritional Information (per serving):
- Calories: 150
- Protein: 2g
- Fat: 7g
- Carbohydrates: 20g
- Fiber: 4g

Lentil and Spinach Soup

Total Time: 45 minutes
Number of Servings: 6

Ingredients:
- 1 cup dried lentils, rinsed

- 6 cups vegetable broth
- 1 onion, diced
- 2 carrots, diced
- 2 celery stalks, diced
- 2 cloves garlic, minced
- 2 cups fresh spinach
- 1 teaspoon ground cumin
- 1 teaspoon dried thyme
- Salt and pepper to taste
- Optional garnish: chopped fresh parsley, lemon wedges

Directions:
1. In a large pot, combine dried lentils and vegetable broth. Bring to a boil, then reduce heat to low and simmer for 20-25 minutes until lentils are tender.
2. In a separate skillet, heat olive oil over medium heat. Add diced onion, carrots, celery, and minced garlic. Sauté for 5-7 minutes until softened.
3. Add sautéed vegetables to the pot of lentils. Stir in fresh spinach, ground cumin, dried thyme, salt, and pepper.
4. Cook for an additional 5-10 minutes until spinach is wilted and flavors are combined.
5. Serve hot, garnished with chopped fresh parsley and lemon wedges if desired.

Nutritional Information (per serving):
- Calories: 200
- Protein: 12g
- Fat: 1g
- Carbohydrates: 35g
- Fiber: 15g

Roasted Butternut Squash Soup

Total Time: 1 hour
Number of Servings: 4

Ingredients:
- 1 butternut squash, peeled, seeded, and cubed
- 1 onion, diced
- 2 cloves garlic, minced
- 4 cups vegetable broth
- 1 teaspoon dried thyme
- 1/2 teaspoon ground cinnamon
- Salt and pepper to taste
- 2 tablespoons olive oil
- Optional garnish: chopped fresh parsley, Greek yogurt

Directions:

1. Preheat the oven to 400°F (200°C). Line a baking sheet with parchment paper.
2. Place cubed butternut squash on the prepared baking sheet. Drizzle with olive oil, and season with salt, pepper, and ground cinnamon. Toss to coat evenly.
3. Roast in the preheated oven for 25-30 minutes until squash is tender and lightly caramelized.
4. In a large pot, heat olive oil over medium heat. Add diced onion and minced garlic. Cook for 5-7 minutes until softened.
5. Add roasted butternut squash cubes to the pot. Pour in vegetable broth and add dried thyme. Bring to a simmer and cook for 15-20 minutes.
6. Use an immersion blender to blend the soup until smooth. Alternatively, transfer the soup to a blender and blend until smooth, then return it to the pot.
7. Season with additional salt and pepper if needed.
8. Serve hot, garnished with chopped fresh parsley and a dollop of Greek yogurt if desired.

Nutritional Information (per serving):

- Calories: 180
- Protein: 3g
- Fat: 7g
- Carbohydrates: 30g
- Fiber: 5g

Chickpea and Kale Soup

Total Time: 40 minutes
Number of Servings: 6

Ingredients:

- 2 tablespoons olive oil
- 1 onion, diced
- 2 carrots, diced
- 2 celery stalks, diced
- 2 cloves garlic, minced
- 1 teaspoon ground cumin
- 1 teaspoon ground coriander
- 1/2 teaspoon smoked paprika
- 4 cups vegetable broth
- 1 can (15 oz) chickpeas, drained and rinsed
- 4 cups chopped kale
- Salt and pepper to taste
- Optional garnish: grated Parmesan cheese, lemon wedges

Directions:

1. Heat olive oil in a large pot over medium heat. Add diced onion, carrots, celery, and minced garlic. Cook for 5-7 minutes until softened.
2. Stir in ground cumin, ground coriander, and smoked paprika. Cook for an additional 2-3 minutes until fragrant.
3. Pour in vegetable broth and bring to a simmer. Add drained and rinsed chickpeas and chopped kale to the pot.
4. Cook for 10-15 minutes until kale is tender.
5. Season with salt and pepper to taste.
6. Serve hot, garnished with grated Parmesan cheese and lemon wedges if desired.

Nutritional Information (per serving):

- Calories: 200
- Protein: 8g
- Fat: 7g
- Carbohydrates: 30g
- Fiber: 8g

Greek Salad with Quinoa

Total Time: 20 minutes
Number of Servings: 4

Ingredients:

- 2 cups cooked quinoa
- 2 cups cherry tomatoes, halved
- 1 cucumber, diced
- 1/2 red onion, thinly sliced
- 1/2 cup Kalamata olives, pitted
- 1/2 cup crumbled feta cheese
- 1/4 cup chopped fresh parsley
- 2 tablespoons olive oil
- 1 tablespoon red wine vinegar
- 1 teaspoon dried oregano
- Salt and pepper to taste

Directions:

1. In a large bowl, combine cooked quinoa, cherry tomatoes, diced cucumber, thinly sliced red onion, pitted Kalamata olives, crumbled feta cheese, and chopped fresh parsley.
2. In a small bowl, whisk together olive oil, red wine vinegar, dried oregano, salt, and pepper.
3. Pour the dressing over the salad ingredients and toss to coat evenly.
4. Serve chilled or at room temperature.

Nutritional Information (per serving):
- Calories: 300
- Protein: 10g
- Fat: 15g
- Carbohydrates: 30g
- Fiber: 5g

Spinach and Strawberry Salad with Walnuts

Total Time: 15 minutes
Number of Servings: 4

Ingredients:
- 6 cups fresh spinach leaves
- 1 cup sliced strawberries
- 1/2 cup chopped walnuts
- 1/4 cup crumbled feta cheese
- Balsamic vinaigrette dressing (store-bought or homemade)

Directions:
1. In a large bowl, combine fresh spinach leaves, sliced strawberries, chopped walnuts, and crumbled feta cheese.
2. Drizzle balsamic vinaigrette dressing over the salad and toss gently to coat evenly.
3. Serve immediately.

Nutritional Information (per serving):
- Calories: 150
- Protein: 5g
- Fat: 10g
- Carbohydrates: 10g
- Fiber: 4g

Beet and Arugula Salad with Goat Cheese

Total Time: 20 minutes
Number of Servings: 4

Ingredients:
- 4 cups baby arugula
- 2 medium beets, roasted and sliced
- 1/4 cup crumbled goat cheese
- 2 tablespoons balsamic vinegar
- 1 tablespoon olive oil

- 1 teaspoon honey
- Salt and pepper to taste

Directions:
1. In a large bowl, combine baby arugula and sliced roasted beets.
2. In a small bowl, whisk together balsamic vinegar, olive oil, honey, salt, and pepper to make the dressing.
3. Drizzle the dressing over the salad and toss gently to coat.
4. Top the salad with crumbled goat cheese before serving.

Nutritional Information (per serving):
- Calories: 120
- Protein: 4g
- Fat: 7g
- Carbohydrates: 12g
- Fiber: 3g

Black Bean and Corn Salad

Total Time: 15 minutes
Number of Servings: 4

Ingredients:
- 1 can (15 oz) black beans, drained and rinsed
- 1 cup frozen corn, thawed
- 1 red bell pepper, diced
- 1/4 cup diced red onion
- 1/4 cup chopped fresh cilantro
- 2 tablespoons lime juice
- 1 tablespoon olive oil
- 1 teaspoon ground cumin
- Salt and pepper to taste

Directions:
1. In a large bowl, combine black beans, thawed corn, diced red bell pepper, diced red onion, and chopped fresh cilantro.
2. In a small bowl, whisk together lime juice, olive oil, ground cumin, salt, and pepper to make the dressing.
3. Pour the dressing over the salad and toss gently to coat.
4. Serve chilled or at room temperature.

Nutritional Information (per serving):
- Calories: 180
- Protein: 7g

- Fat: 4g
- Carbohydrates: 30g
- Fiber: 8g

Mixed Greens with Berries and Almonds

Total Time: 15 minutes
Number of Servings: 4

Ingredients:
- 6 cups mixed salad greens (such as spinach, arugula, and lettuce)
- 1 cup mixed berries (such as strawberries, blueberries, and raspberries)
- 1/4 cup sliced almonds
- Balsamic vinaigrette dressing (store-bought or homemade)

Directions:
1. In a large bowl, combine mixed salad greens, mixed berries, and sliced almonds.
2. Drizzle balsamic vinaigrette dressing over the salad and toss gently to coat evenly.
3. Serve immediately.

Nutritional Information (per serving):
- Calories: 120
- Protein: 5g
- Fat: 7g
- Carbohydrates: 15g
- Fiber: 6g

Broccoli and Apple Salad with Greek Yogurt Dressing

Total Time: 20 minutes
Number of Servings: 4

Ingredients:
- 4 cups broccoli florets
- 1 large apple, diced
- 1/4 cup dried cranberries
- 1/4 cup chopped pecans
- 1/2 cup plain Greek yogurt
- 2 tablespoons apple cider vinegar
- 1 tablespoon honey
- Salt and pepper to taste

Directions:

1. In a large bowl, combine broccoli florets, diced apple, dried cranberries, and chopped pecans.
2. In a small bowl, whisk together plain Greek yogurt, apple cider vinegar, honey, salt, and pepper to make the dressing.
3. Pour the dressing over the salad and toss gently to coat.
4. Serve chilled or at room temperature.

Nutritional Information (per serving):

- Calories: 150
- Protein: 6g
- Fat: 5g
- Carbohydrates: 25g
- Fiber: 6g

Fish and Seafood

Grilled Salmon with Quinoa and Steamed Spinach

Total Time: 30 minutes
Number of Servings: 4

Ingredients:
- 4 salmon fillets
- 1 cup quinoa
- 2 cups water or vegetable broth
- 4 cups fresh spinach leaves
- Olive oil
- Salt and pepper to taste
- Lemon wedges for serving

Directions:
1. Cook quinoa according to package instructions using water or vegetable broth.
2. Preheat grill to medium-high heat.
3. Season salmon fillets with salt, pepper, and a drizzle of olive oil.
4. Grill salmon for 4-5 minutes per side, or until cooked through and flaky.
5. While salmon is grilling, steam fresh spinach until wilted.
6. Serve grilled salmon over cooked quinoa with steamed spinach on the side.
7. Garnish with lemon wedges and serve hot.

Nutritional Information (per serving):
- Calories: 350
- Protein: 30g
- Fat: 15g
- Carbohydrates: 20g
- Fiber: 4g

Baked Cod with Garlic and Lemon

Total Time: 25 minutes
Number of Servings: 4

Ingredients:
- 4 cod fillets
- 2 cloves garlic, minced
- 2 tablespoons olive oil
- 1 lemon, sliced

- Salt and pepper to taste
- Fresh parsley for garnish

Directions:
1. Preheat oven to 400°F (200°C).
2. Place cod fillets on a baking sheet lined with parchment paper.
3. In a small bowl, mix minced garlic with olive oil. Drizzle the garlic mixture over the cod fillets.
4. Season cod fillets with salt and pepper. Place lemon slices on top of each fillet.
5. Bake in the preheated oven for 15-20 minutes, or until fish is cooked through and flakes easily with a fork.
6. Garnish with fresh parsley before serving.

Nutritional Information (per serving):
- Calories: 200
- Protein: 25g
- Fat: 8g
- Carbohydrates: 2g
- Fiber: 1g

Shrimp and Avocado Salad

Total Time: 20 minutes
Number of Servings: 4

Ingredients:
- 1 lb cooked shrimp, peeled and deveined
- 2 avocados, diced
- 1 cup cherry tomatoes, halved
- 1/4 cup chopped cilantro
- 1/4 cup diced red onion
- Juice of 1 lime
- 2 tablespoons olive oil
- Salt and pepper to taste

Directions:
1. In a large bowl, combine cooked shrimp, diced avocados, halved cherry tomatoes, chopped cilantro, and diced red onion.
2. Drizzle lime juice and olive oil over the salad. Season with salt and pepper to taste.
3. Toss gently to combine all ingredients.
4. Serve chilled or at room temperature.

Nutritional Information (per serving):
- Calories: 250

- Protein: 20g
- Fat: 15g
- Carbohydrates: 10g
- Fiber: 6g

Tuna and White Bean Salad

Total Time: 15 minutes
Number of Servings: 4

Ingredients:
- 2 cans (5 oz each) tuna, drained
- 1 can (15 oz) white beans, drained and rinsed
- 1/4 cup chopped red onion
- 1/4 cup chopped parsley
- 2 tablespoons olive oil
- 1 tablespoon red wine vinegar
- Salt and pepper to taste

Directions:
1. In a large bowl, combine drained tuna, white beans, chopped red onion, and chopped parsley.
2. Drizzle olive oil and red wine vinegar over the salad. Season with salt and pepper to taste.
3. Toss gently to combine all ingredients.
4. Serve chilled or at room temperature.

Nutritional Information (per serving):
- Calories: 300
- Protein: 25g
- Fat: 10g
- Carbohydrates: 20g
- Fiber: 6g

Salmon Burgers with Whole Grain Bun

Total Time: 20 minutes
Number of Servings: 4

Ingredients:
- 1 lb salmon fillets, skin removed
- 1/4 cup breadcrumbs
- 1 egg
- 2 green onions, finely chopped

- 1 tablespoon Dijon mustard
- 1 tablespoon lemon juice
- Salt and pepper to taste
- 4 whole grain burger buns
- Optional toppings: lettuce, tomato, avocado, Greek yogurt

Directions:
1. In a food processor, pulse salmon fillets until finely chopped.
2. In a large bowl, combine chopped salmon, breadcrumbs, egg, chopped green onions, Dijon mustard, lemon juice, salt, and pepper.
3. Divide the salmon mixture into 4 equal portions and shape into burger patties.
4. Heat olive oil in a skillet over medium heat. Cook salmon burgers for 3-4 minutes per side, or until cooked through.
5. Toast whole grain burger buns on a grill or in the oven.
6. Assemble the burgers by placing a salmon patty on each bun. Add desired toppings such as lettuce, tomato, avocado, and Greek yogurt.
7. Serve hot.

Nutritional Information (per serving):
- Calories: 350
- Protein: 30g
- Fat: 15g
- Carbohydrates: 25g
- Fiber: 5g

Baked Tilapia with Herbs and Brown Rice

Total Time: 30 minutes
Number of Servings: 4

Ingredients:
- 4 tilapia fillets
- 2 tablespoons olive oil
- 2 cloves garlic, minced
- 1 tablespoon chopped fresh parsley
- 1 tablespoon chopped fresh dill
- 1 lemon, sliced
- Salt and pepper to taste
- 2 cups cooked brown rice

Directions:
1. Preheat the oven to 400°F (200°C). Line a baking sheet with parchment paper.
2. Place tilapia fillets on the prepared baking sheet.

3. In a small bowl, mix together olive oil, minced garlic, chopped fresh parsley, and chopped fresh dill. Drizzle the mixture over the tilapia fillets.
4. Place lemon slices on top of each fillet. Season with salt and pepper.
5. Bake in the preheated oven for 15-20 minutes, or until fish is cooked through and flakes easily with a fork.
6. Serve baked tilapia over cooked brown rice.

Nutritional Information (per serving):
- Calories: 250
- Protein: 25g
- Fat: 10g
- Carbohydrates: 15g
- Fiber: 2g

Grilled Mackerel with Tomato Salsa

Total Time: 25 minutes
Number of Servings: 4

Ingredients:
- 4 mackerel fillets
- 2 tablespoons olive oil
- 1 teaspoon smoked paprika
- 1 teaspoon ground cumin
- Salt and pepper to taste
- For Tomato Salsa:
    - 2 tomatoes, diced
    - 1/4 cup diced red onion
    - 1/4 cup chopped fresh cilantro
    - Juice of 1 lime
    - Salt and pepper to taste

Directions:
1. Preheat grill to medium-high heat.
2. Brush mackerel fillets with olive oil. Season with smoked paprika, ground cumin, salt, and pepper.
3. Grill mackerel fillets for 4-5 minutes per side, or until cooked through and charred.
4. In a bowl, combine diced tomatoes, diced red onion, chopped fresh cilantro, lime juice, salt, and pepper to make the tomato salsa.
5. Serve grilled mackerel fillets with tomato salsa on top.

Nutritional Information (per serving):
- Calories: 280
- Protein: 30g

- Fat: 15g
- Carbohydrates: 5g
- Fiber: 2g

Fish Tacos with Cabbage Slaw

Total Time: 30 minutes
Number of Servings: 4

Ingredients:
- 1 lb white fish fillets (such as cod or tilapia)
- 2 tablespoons olive oil
- 1 tablespoon chili powder
- 1 teaspoon ground cumin
- 1 teaspoon smoked paprika
- Salt and pepper to taste
- 8 small corn tortillas
- For Cabbage Slaw:
    - 2 cups shredded cabbage
    - 1/4 cup chopped fresh cilantro
    - 2 tablespoons Greek yogurt
    - 1 tablespoon lime juice
    - Salt and pepper to taste

Directions:
1. Preheat the oven to 400°F (200°C). Line a baking sheet with parchment paper.
2. Brush fish fillets with olive oil. Season with chili powder, ground cumin, smoked paprika, salt, and pepper.
3. Bake fish fillets in the preheated oven for 15-20 minutes, or until fish is cooked through and flakes easily with a fork.
4. While the fish is baking, prepare the cabbage slaw. In a bowl, combine shredded cabbage, chopped fresh cilantro, Greek yogurt, lime juice, salt, and pepper. Toss to coat evenly.
5. Warm corn tortillas in a skillet over medium heat.
6. Assemble fish tacos by placing baked fish fillets on warm corn tortillas and topping with cabbage slaw.
7. Serve hot.

Nutritional Information (per serving):
- Calories: 300
- Protein: 25g
- Fat: 10g
- Carbohydrates: 25g
- Fiber: 4g

Spicy Shrimp Stir-Fry with Vegetables

Total Time: 20 minutes
Number of Servings: 4

Ingredients:
- 1 lb large shrimp, peeled and deveined
- 2 tablespoons olive oil
- 2 cloves garlic, minced
- 1 teaspoon grated ginger
- 1 bell pepper, sliced
- 1 cup broccoli florets
- 1 cup sliced mushrooms
- 1/4 cup soy sauce
- 2 tablespoons Sriracha sauce (adjust to taste)
- 2 green onions, sliced
- Cooked rice or quinoa for serving

Directions:
1. Heat olive oil in a large skillet or wok over medium-high heat.
2. Add minced garlic and grated ginger to the skillet. Stir-fry for 1 minute until fragrant.
3. Add bell pepper, broccoli florets, and sliced mushrooms to the skillet. Stir-fry for 3-4 minutes until vegetables are tender-crisp.
4. Push vegetables to the side of the skillet and add shrimp. Cook shrimp for 2-3 minutes until pink and cooked through.
5. In a small bowl, mix together soy sauce and Sriracha sauce. Pour the sauce over the shrimp and vegetables. Stir to coat evenly.
6. Add sliced green onions to the skillet and toss to combine.
7. Serve spicy shrimp stir-fry over cooked rice or quinoa.

Nutritional Information (per serving):
- Calories: 250
- Protein: 25g
- Fat: 10g
- Carbohydrates: 15g
- Fiber: 3g

Tuna Steak with Quinoa and Asparagus

Total Time: 30 minutes
Number of Servings: 4

Ingredients:
- 4 tuna steaks
- 2 tablespoons olive oil
- 2 cloves garlic, minced
- 1 teaspoon lemon zest
- Salt and pepper to taste
- 2 cups cooked quinoa
- 1 lb asparagus, trimmed
- Lemon wedges for serving

Directions:
1. Preheat grill or grill pan to medium-high heat.
2. Brush tuna steaks with olive oil. Season with minced garlic, lemon zest, salt, and pepper.
3. Grill tuna steaks for 3-4 minutes per side, or until desired doneness.
4. While the tuna is grilling, steam asparagus until tender.
5. Serve grilled tuna steaks with cooked quinoa and steamed asparagus.
6. Garnish with lemon wedges and serve hot.

Nutritional Information (per serving):
- Calories: 300
- Protein: 35g
- Fat: 10g
- Carbohydrates: 20g
- Fiber: 5g

Grains and Legumes

Quinoa Salad with Black Beans and Corn

Total Time: 20 minutes
Number of Servings: 4

Ingredients:
- 1 cup quinoa
- 2 cups water or vegetable broth
- 1 can (15 oz) black beans, drained and rinsed
- 1 cup corn kernels (fresh or frozen)
- 1 red bell pepper, diced
- 1/4 cup chopped fresh cilantro
- Juice of 1 lime
- 2 tablespoons olive oil
- Salt and pepper to taste
- Optional toppings: avocado, diced tomatoes, crumbled feta cheese

Directions:
1. Rinse quinoa under cold water. In a saucepan, combine quinoa and water or vegetable broth. Bring to a boil, then reduce heat to low, cover, and simmer for 15 minutes, or until quinoa is cooked and liquid is absorbed.
2. In a large bowl, combine cooked quinoa, black beans, corn kernels, diced red bell pepper, and chopped fresh cilantro.
3. In a small bowl, whisk together lime juice, olive oil, salt, and pepper to make the dressing.
4. Pour the dressing over the quinoa salad and toss gently to coat all ingredients.
5. Serve quinoa salad at room temperature or chilled, topped with optional toppings if desired.

Nutritional Information (per serving):
- Calories: 300
- Protein: 10g
- Fat: 8g
- Carbohydrates: 50g
- Fiber: 10g

Brown Rice Pilaf with Vegetables

Total Time: 40 minutes
Number of Servings: 4

Ingredients:
- 1 cup brown rice
- 2 cups water or vegetable broth
- 1 tablespoon olive oil
- 1 onion, diced
- 2 cloves garlic, minced
- 2 carrots, diced
- 1 red bell pepper, diced
- 1 cup frozen peas
- 1/4 cup chopped fresh parsley
- Salt and pepper to taste

Directions:
1. Rinse brown rice under cold water. In a saucepan, combine brown rice and water or vegetable broth. Bring to a boil, then reduce heat to low, cover, and simmer for 30-35 minutes, or until rice is tender and liquid is absorbed.
2. In a large skillet, heat olive oil over medium heat. Add diced onion and minced garlic. Cook for 2-3 minutes until softened and fragrant.
3. Add diced carrots and diced red bell pepper to the skillet. Cook for 5-7 minutes until vegetables are tender.
4. Stir in cooked brown rice and frozen peas. Cook for an additional 3-4 minutes until heated through.
5. Season with chopped fresh parsley, salt, and pepper.
6. Serve brown rice pilaf hot as a side dish or a main course.

Nutritional Information (per serving):
- Calories: 250
- Protein: 5g
- Fat: 5g
- Carbohydrates: 45g
- Fiber: 7g

Lentil and Vegetable Stew

Total Time: 45 minutes
Number of Servings: 6

Ingredients:
- 1 cup dried green lentils
- 4 cups vegetable broth
- 2 tablespoons olive oil
- 1 onion, diced
- 2 carrots, diced
- 2 stalks celery, diced
- 2 cloves garlic, minced
- 1 can (14 oz) diced tomatoes
- 2 cups chopped spinach
- 1 teaspoon dried thyme
- 1 teaspoon dried rosemary
- Salt and pepper to taste

Directions:
1. Rinse dried green lentils under cold water. In a large pot, combine lentils and vegetable broth. Bring to a boil, then reduce heat to low, cover, and simmer for 20-25 minutes, or until lentils are tender.
2. In a separate skillet, heat olive oil over medium heat. Add diced onion, diced carrots, diced celery, and minced garlic. Cook for 5-7 minutes until vegetables are softened.
3. Add cooked vegetables to the pot of lentils. Stir in diced tomatoes, chopped spinach, dried thyme, dried rosemary, salt, and pepper.
4. Simmer the stew for an additional 10-15 minutes to allow flavors to blend.
5. Adjust seasoning if needed and serve hot.

Nutritional Information (per serving):
- Calories: 200
- Protein: 10g
- Fat: 5g
- Carbohydrates: 30g
- Fiber: 10g

Barley and Mushroom Risotto

Total Time: 45 minutes
Number of Servings: 4

Ingredients:
- 1 cup pearl barley
- 4 cups vegetable broth
- 2 tablespoons olive oil
- 1 onion, diced
- 2 cloves garlic, minced
- 8 oz mushrooms, sliced
- 1/4 cup grated Parmesan cheese
- Salt and pepper to taste
- Chopped fresh parsley for garnish

Directions:
1. Rinse pearl barley under cold water. In a saucepan, combine barley and vegetable broth. Bring to a boil, then reduce heat to low, cover, and simmer for 30-35 minutes, or until barley is tender and liquid is absorbed.
2. In a separate skillet, heat olive oil over medium heat. Add diced onion and minced garlic. Cook for 2-3 minutes until softened and fragrant.
3. Add sliced mushrooms to the skillet. Cook for 5-7 minutes until mushrooms are tender and golden brown.
4. Stir cooked mushrooms into the pot of barley. Mix in grated Parmesan cheese. Season with salt and pepper.
5. Garnish with chopped fresh parsley before serving.

Nutritional Information (per serving):
- Calories: 250
- Protein: 8g
- Fat: 7g
- Carbohydrates: 40g
- Fiber: 8g

Chickpea and Spinach Curry

Total Time: 30 minutes
Number of Servings: 4

Ingredients:
- 1 tablespoon olive oil
- 1 onion, diced

- 2 cloves garlic, minced
- 1 tablespoon grated ginger
- 1 tablespoon curry powder
- 1 teaspoon ground cumin
- 1 can (15 oz) chickpeas, drained and rinsed
- 1 can (14 oz) diced tomatoes
- 2 cups chopped spinach
- 1/2 cup coconut milk
- Salt and pepper to taste
- Cooked rice for serving

Directions:
1. Heat olive oil in a large skillet over medium heat. Add diced onion, minced garlic, and grated ginger. Cook for 2-3 minutes until softened and fragrant.
2. Stir in curry powder and ground cumin. Cook for an additional 1-2 minutes until spices are toasted.
3. Add drained chickpeas and diced tomatoes to the skillet. Simmer for 10-15 minutes, stirring occasionally.
4. Stir in chopped spinach and coconut milk. Cook for an additional 3-5 minutes until spinach is wilted.
5. Season with salt and pepper to taste.
6. Serve chickpea and spinach curry over cooked rice.

Nutritional Information (per serving):
- Calories: 300
- Protein: 10g
- Fat: 10g
- Carbohydrates: 45g
- Fiber: 10g

Farro Salad with Cherry Tomatoes and Basil

Total Time: 30 minutes
Number of Servings: 4

Ingredients:
- 1 cup farro
- 2 cups water or vegetable broth
- 1 pint cherry tomatoes, halved
- 1/4 cup chopped fresh basil
- 2 tablespoons olive oil
- 1 tablespoon balsamic vinegar
- Salt and pepper to taste
- Optional: crumbled feta cheese or diced avocado for topping

Directions:
1. Rinse farro under cold water. In a saucepan, combine farro and water or vegetable broth. Bring to a boil, then reduce heat to low, cover, and simmer for 20-25 minutes, or until farro is tender.
2. In a large bowl, combine cooked farro, halved cherry tomatoes, and chopped fresh basil.
3. In a small bowl, whisk together olive oil, balsamic vinegar, salt, and pepper to make the dressing.
4. Pour the dressing over the farro salad and toss gently to coat all ingredients.
5. Serve farro salad at room temperature or chilled, topped with optional toppings if desired.

Nutritional Information (per serving):
- Calories: 250
- Protein: 6g
- Fat: 8g
- Carbohydrates: 40g
- Fiber: 8g

Black Bean and Sweet Potato Enchiladas

Total Time: 45 minutes
Number of Servings: 4

Ingredients:
- 1 tablespoon olive oil
- 1 onion, diced
- 2 cloves garlic, minced
- 1 sweet potato, peeled and diced
- 1 can (15 oz) black beans, drained and rinsed
- 1 teaspoon chili powder
- 1 teaspoon ground cumin
- Salt and pepper to taste
- 8 small whole wheat tortillas
- 1 cup enchilada sauce
- 1/2 cup shredded cheddar cheese or vegan cheese
- Chopped fresh cilantro for garnish

Directions:
1. Preheat the oven to 375°F (190°C).
2. Heat olive oil in a large skillet over medium heat. Add diced onion and minced garlic. Cook for 2-3 minutes until softened and fragrant.
3. Add diced sweet potato to the skillet. Cook for 5-7 minutes until sweet potato is tender.
4. Stir in drained black beans, chili powder, ground cumin, salt, and pepper. Cook for an additional 2-3 minutes to heat through.

5. Place a spoonful of the black bean and sweet potato mixture onto each whole wheat tortilla. Roll up the tortillas and place them seam-side down in a baking dish.
6. Pour enchilada sauce over the rolled tortillas. Sprinkle shredded cheddar cheese or vegan cheese on top.
7. Bake in the preheated oven for 20-25 minutes, or until cheese is melted and bubbly.
8. Garnish with chopped fresh cilantro before serving.

Nutritional Information (per serving):
- Calories: 350
- Protein: 12g
- Fat: 10g
- Carbohydrates: 55g
- Fiber: 12g

Lentil Soup with Carrots and Celery

Total Time: 40 minutes
Number of Servings: 6

Ingredients:
- 1 cup dried green or brown lentils
- 6 cups vegetable broth
- 1 tablespoon olive oil
- 1 onion, diced
- 2 carrots, diced
- 2 stalks celery, diced
- 2 cloves garlic, minced
- 1 teaspoon dried thyme
- 1 teaspoon dried rosemary
- Salt and pepper to taste
- Chopped fresh parsley for garnish

Directions:
1. Rinse dried lentils under cold water. In a large pot, combine lentils and vegetable broth. Bring to a boil, then reduce heat to low, cover, and simmer for 20-25 minutes, or until lentils are tender.
2. In a separate skillet, heat olive oil over medium heat. Add diced onion, diced carrots, diced celery, and minced garlic. Cook for 5-7 minutes until vegetables are softened.
3. Add cooked vegetables to the pot of lentils. Stir in dried thyme, dried rosemary, salt, and pepper.
4. Simmer the lentil soup for an additional 10-15 minutes to allow flavors to blend.
5. Adjust seasoning if needed and serve hot, garnished with chopped fresh parsley.

Nutritional Information (per serving):
- Calories: 250
- Protein: 12g
- Fat: 5g
- Carbohydrates: 40g
- Fiber: 12g

Bulgur Wheat Salad with Pomegranate

Total Time: 25 minutes
Number of Servings: 4

Ingredients:
- 1 cup bulgur wheat
- 2 cups water or vegetable broth
- 1/2 cup pomegranate arils
- 1/4 cup chopped fresh mint
- 1/4 cup chopped fresh parsley
- 2 tablespoons olive oil
- 1 tablespoon lemon juice
- Salt and pepper to taste
- Optional: crumbled feta cheese or diced cucumber for topping

Directions:
1. Rinse bulgur wheat under cold water. In a saucepan, combine bulgur wheat and water or vegetable broth. Bring to a boil, then reduce heat to low, cover, and simmer for 10-12 minutes, or until bulgur wheat is tender.
2. In a large bowl, combine cooked bulgur wheat, pomegranate arils, chopped fresh mint, and chopped fresh parsley.
3. In a small bowl, whisk together olive oil, lemon juice, salt, and pepper to make the dressing.
4. Pour the dressing over the bulgur wheat salad and toss gently to coat all ingredients.
5. Serve bulgur wheat salad at room temperature or chilled, topped with optional toppings if desired.

Nutritional Information (per serving):
- Calories: 200
- Protein: 5g
- Fat: 7g
- Carbohydrates: 30g
- Fiber: 8g

Red Lentil Dal with Brown Rice

Total Time: 35 minutes
Number of Servings: 4

Ingredients:
- 1 cup dried red lentils
- 4 cups water or vegetable broth
- 1 tablespoon olive oil
- 1 onion, diced
- 2 cloves garlic, minced
- 1 teaspoon grated ginger
- 1 teaspoon ground cumin
- 1 teaspoon ground turmeric
- 1/2 teaspoon ground coriander
- Salt and pepper to taste
- Cooked brown rice for serving
- Chopped fresh cilantro for garnish

Directions:
1. Rinse dried red lentils under cold water. In a large pot, combine red lentils and water or vegetable broth. Bring to a boil, then reduce heat to low, cover, and simmer for 20-25 minutes, or until lentils are soft and cooked through.
2. In a separate skillet, heat olive oil over medium heat. Add diced onion, minced garlic, and grated ginger. Cook for 2-3 minutes until softened and fragrant.
3. Stir in ground cumin, ground turmeric, and ground coriander. Cook for an additional 1-2 minutes until spices are toasted.
4. Add cooked lentils to the skillet. Stir to combine with the onion and spice mixture. If the dal is too thick, you can add more water or vegetable broth to reach your desired consistency.
5. Season with salt and pepper to taste.
6. Serve red lentil dal over cooked brown rice, garnished with chopped fresh cilantro.

Nutritional Information (per serving):
- Calories: 300
- Protein: 15g
- Fat: 5g
- Carbohydrates: 50g
- Fiber: 10g

Nuts and Seeds

Almond and Berry Smoothie

Total Time: 5 minutes
Number of Servings: 2

Ingredients:
- 1 cup almond milk
- 1 ripe banana
- 1/2 cup mixed berries (such as strawberries, blueberries, raspberries)
- 2 tablespoons almond butter
- 1 tablespoon chia seeds
- Optional: honey or maple syrup to sweeten

Directions:
1. In a blender, combine almond milk, ripe banana, mixed berries, almond butter, and chia seeds.
2. Blend until smooth and creamy.
3. Taste and adjust sweetness with honey or maple syrup if desired.
4. Pour into glasses and serve immediately.

Nutritional Information (per serving):
- Calories: 200
- Protein: 5g
- Fat: 10g
- Carbohydrates: 25g
- Fiber: 7g

Chia Seed Pudding with Almond Milk

Total Time: 4 hours (including chilling time)
Number of Servings: 4

Ingredients:
- 1/2 cup chia seeds
- 2 cups almond milk
- 1 teaspoon vanilla extract
- 1 tablespoon maple syrup or honey
- Optional toppings: fresh berries, sliced almonds, shredded coconut

Directions:

1. In a mixing bowl, combine chia seeds, almond milk, vanilla extract, and maple syrup or honey. Stir well to combine.
2. Cover the bowl and refrigerate for at least 4 hours or overnight, until the chia seeds have absorbed the liquid and the mixture has thickened to a pudding-like consistency.
3. Stir the chia seed pudding before serving to evenly distribute the seeds.
4. Serve chilled, topped with fresh berries, sliced almonds, or shredded coconut if desired.

Nutritional Information (per serving):

- Calories: 150
- Protein: 4g
- Fat: 8g
- Carbohydrates: 15g
- Fiber: 8g

Quinoa Salad with Pumpkin Seeds

Total Time: 20 minutes
Number of Servings: 4

Ingredients:

- 1 cup cooked quinoa
- 1/2 cup diced cucumber
- 1/2 cup diced bell pepper
- 1/4 cup chopped fresh parsley
- 2 tablespoons lemon juice
- 2 tablespoons olive oil
- Salt and pepper to taste
- 1/4 cup pumpkin seeds (pepitas)

Directions:

1. In a large bowl, combine cooked quinoa, diced cucumber, diced bell pepper, and chopped fresh parsley.
2. In a small bowl, whisk together lemon juice, olive oil, salt, and pepper to make the dressing.
3. Pour the dressing over the quinoa salad and toss gently to coat all ingredients.
4. Sprinkle pumpkin seeds over the salad before serving.

Nutritional Information (per serving):

- Calories: 200
- Protein: 5g
- Fat: 10g
- Carbohydrates: 20g
- Fiber: 5g

Spinach and Walnut Pesto Pasta

Total Time: 20 minutes
Number of Servings: 4

Ingredients:
- 8 oz whole wheat spaghetti or pasta of your choice
- 2 cups fresh spinach leaves
- 1/2 cup walnuts
- 2 cloves garlic
- 1/4 cup grated Parmesan cheese
- 1/4 cup olive oil
- Salt and pepper to taste

Directions:
1. Cook pasta according to package instructions. Drain and set aside.
2. In a food processor, combine fresh spinach leaves, walnuts, garlic, and grated Parmesan cheese. Pulse until coarsely chopped.
3. With the food processor running, slowly drizzle in olive oil until the pesto reaches your desired consistency. Season with salt and pepper to taste.
4. Toss cooked pasta with the spinach and walnut pesto until well coated.
5. Serve hot, garnished with additional grated Parmesan cheese if desired.

Nutritional Information (per serving):
- Calories: 350
- Protein: 10g
- Fat: 20g
- Carbohydrates: 30g
- Fiber: 5g

Mixed Nut and Seed Energy Bars

Total Time: 30 minutes
Number of Servings: 8 bars

Ingredients:
- 1 cup mixed nuts (such as almonds, cashews, peanuts)
- 1/2 cup mixed seeds (such as pumpkin seeds, sunflower seeds, chia seeds)
- 1/2 cup rolled oats
- 1/4 cup honey or maple syrup
- 1/4 cup almond butter or peanut butter
- 1/2 teaspoon vanilla extract
- Pinch of salt

Directions:
1. Preheat the oven to 350°F (175°C). Line a baking dish with parchment paper.
2. In a food processor, pulse mixed nuts, mixed seeds, and rolled oats until coarsely chopped.
3. In a small saucepan, combine honey or maple syrup, almond butter or peanut butter, vanilla extract, and a pinch of salt. Heat over low heat until melted and well combined.
4. Pour the melted nut butter mixture over the chopped nuts, seeds, and oats. Stir until everything is evenly coated.
5. Press the mixture into the prepared baking dish in an even layer.
6. Bake in the preheated oven for 15-20 minutes, or until the edges are golden brown.
7. Remove from the oven and let cool completely in the baking dish.
8. Once cooled, cut into bars or squares.

Nutritional Information (per serving):
- Calories: 200
- Protein: 5g
- Fat: 12g
- Carbohydrates: 20g
- Fiber: 4g

Flaxseed and Banana Smoothie

Total Time: 5 minutes
Number of Servings: 2

Ingredients:
- 1 ripe banana
- 1 tablespoon ground flaxseed
- 1 cup almond milk (or milk of your choice)
- 1/2 cup Greek yogurt
- 1 tablespoon honey (optional)
- Handful of ice cubes

Directions:
1. Peel the banana and break it into chunks.
2. In a blender, combine the banana chunks, ground flaxseed, almond milk, Greek yogurt, honey (if using), and ice cubes.
3. Blend until smooth and creamy.
4. Pour into glasses and serve immediately.

Nutritional Information (per serving):
- Calories: 150
- Protein: 6g
- Fat: 4g

- Carbohydrates: 25g
- Fiber: 5g

Spinach Salad with Sunflower Seeds

Total Time: 10 minutes
Number of Servings: 2

Ingredients:
- 4 cups fresh spinach leaves
- 1/4 cup sunflower seeds
- 1/2 cup cherry tomatoes, halved
- 1/4 cup sliced red onion
- 2 tablespoons balsamic vinaigrette dressing

Directions:
1. In a large bowl, combine fresh spinach leaves, sunflower seeds, cherry tomatoes, and sliced red onion.
2. Drizzle balsamic vinaigrette dressing over the salad.
3. Toss gently to coat all ingredients.
4. Serve immediately.

Nutritional Information (per serving):
- Calories: 100
- Protein: 4g
- Fat: 7g
- Carbohydrates: 8g
- Fiber: 3g

Almond Crusted Chicken

Total Time: 25 minutes
Number of Servings: 4

Ingredients:
- 4 boneless, skinless chicken breasts
- 1/2 cup almond meal or ground almonds
- 1/4 cup grated Parmesan cheese
- 1 teaspoon garlic powder
- 1 teaspoon paprika
- Salt and pepper to taste
- 1 egg, beaten
- 2 tablespoons olive oil

Directions:
1. Preheat the oven to 400°F (200°C). Grease a baking sheet with olive oil or line it with parchment paper.
2. In a shallow bowl, combine almond meal, grated Parmesan cheese, garlic powder, paprika, salt, and pepper.
3. Dip each chicken breast into the beaten egg, then dredge it in the almond meal mixture, pressing gently to coat both sides.
4. Place the coated chicken breasts on the prepared baking sheet.
5. Drizzle olive oil over the top of each chicken breast.
6. Bake in the preheated oven for 20-25 minutes, or until the chicken is cooked through and the crust is golden brown.
7. Serve hot.

Nutritional Information (per serving):
- Calories: 250
- Protein: 30g
- Fat: 12g
- Carbohydrates: 5g
- Fiber: 2g

Chia and Flaxseed Granola

Total Time: 30 minutes
Number of Servings: 8

Ingredients:
- 2 cups rolled oats
- 1/2 cup unsweetened shredded coconut
- 1/4 cup chia seeds
- 1/4 cup ground flaxseed
- 1/4 cup honey or maple syrup
- 1/4 cup coconut oil, melted
- 1 teaspoon vanilla extract
- Pinch of salt
- 1/2 cup dried fruit (such as raisins, cranberries, or chopped apricots)
- 1/4 cup nuts or seeds (such as almonds, walnuts, or pumpkin seeds)

Directions:
1. Preheat the oven to 300°F (150°C). Line a baking sheet with parchment paper.
2. In a large bowl, combine rolled oats, shredded coconut, chia seeds, ground flaxseed, honey or maple syrup, melted coconut oil, vanilla extract, and a pinch of salt. Mix well to combine.
3. Spread the granola mixture evenly onto the prepared baking sheet.

4. Bake in the preheated oven for 20-25 minutes, stirring occasionally, until the granola is golden brown and crispy.
5. Remove from the oven and let cool completely.
6. Once cooled, stir in dried fruit and nuts or seeds.
7. Store the granola in an airtight container at room temperature for up to two weeks.

Nutritional Information (per serving):
- Calories: 200
- Protein: 5g
- Fat: 10g
- Carbohydrates: 25g
- Fiber: 5g

Roasted Pumpkin Seeds Snack

Total Time: 45 minutes
Number of Servings: 4

Ingredients:
- 1 cup raw pumpkin seeds (pepitas)
- 1 tablespoon olive oil
- 1 teaspoon salt
- Optional seasonings: garlic powder, onion powder, chili powder, cayenne pepper

Directions:
1. Preheat the oven to 300°F (150°C). Line a baking sheet with parchment paper.
2. In a bowl, toss pumpkin seeds with olive oil and salt until evenly coated.
3. Spread the pumpkin seeds in a single layer on the prepared baking sheet.
4. Bake in the preheated oven for 30-40 minutes, stirring occasionally, until the pumpkin seeds are golden brown and crispy.
5. Remove from the oven and let cool before serving.
6. Optional: Season with additional spices like garlic powder, onion powder, chili powder, or cayenne pepper for extra flavor.

Nutritional Information (per serving):
- Calories: 160
- Protein: 8g
- Fat: 14g
- Carbohydrates: 3g
- Fiber: 2g

Side and Savory Snack

Roasted Brussels Sprouts with Balsamic Glaze

Total Time: 30 minutes
Number of Servings: 4

Ingredients:
- 1 lb Brussels sprouts, trimmed and halved
- 2 tablespoons olive oil
- Salt and pepper to taste
- 2 tablespoons balsamic glaze

Directions:
1. Preheat the oven to 400°F (200°C).
2. In a large bowl, toss Brussels sprouts with olive oil, salt, and pepper until evenly coated.
3. Spread Brussels sprouts in a single layer on a baking sheet.
4. Roast in the preheated oven for 20-25 minutes, or until Brussels sprouts are tender and caramelized.
5. Drizzle with balsamic glaze before serving.

Nutritional Information (per serving):
- Calories: 100
- Protein: 4g
- Fat: 5g
- Carbohydrates: 12g
- Fiber: 4g

Sweet Potato Fries with Paprika

Total Time: 40 minutes
Number of Servings: 4

Ingredients:
- 2 large sweet potatoes, peeled and cut into fries
- 2 tablespoons olive oil
- 1 teaspoon paprika
- Salt and pepper to taste

Directions:
1. Preheat the oven to 425°F (220°C).

2. In a large bowl, toss sweet potato fries with olive oil, paprika, salt, and pepper until evenly coated.
3. Spread sweet potato fries in a single layer on a baking sheet lined with parchment paper.
4. Bake in the preheated oven for 25-30 minutes, flipping halfway through, or until fries are crispy and golden brown.
5. Serve hot.

Nutritional Information (per serving):
- Calories: 150
- Protein: 2g
- Fat: 7g
- Carbohydrates: 20g
- Fiber: 4g

Steamed Broccoli with Lemon and Garlic

Total Time: 15 minutes
Number of Servings: 4

Ingredients:
- 1 lb broccoli florets
- 2 cloves garlic, minced
- Zest and juice of 1 lemon
- Salt and pepper to taste

Directions:
1. Place broccoli florets in a steamer basket over a pot of boiling water.
2. Cover and steam for 5-7 minutes, or until broccoli is tender but still crisp.
3. In a small saucepan, heat a bit of olive oil over medium heat. Add minced garlic and cook for 1-2 minutes until fragrant.
4. Remove steamed broccoli from the steamer basket and transfer to a serving bowl.
5. Drizzle with the garlic-infused olive oil, lemon zest, and lemon juice. Season with salt and pepper to taste.
6. Toss gently to coat broccoli with the dressing before serving.

Nutritional Information (per serving):
- Calories: 50
- Protein: 3g
- Fat: 1g
- Carbohydrates: 10g
- Fiber: 4g

Roasted Cauliflower with Turmeric

Total Time: 25 minutes
Number of Servings: 4

Ingredients:
- 1 head cauliflower, cut into florets
- 2 tablespoons olive oil
- 1 teaspoon ground turmeric
- Salt and pepper to taste

Directions:
1. Preheat the oven to 425°F (220°C).
2. In a large bowl, toss cauliflower florets with olive oil, ground turmeric, salt, and pepper until evenly coated.
3. Spread cauliflower florets in a single layer on a baking sheet lined with parchment paper.
4. Roast in the preheated oven for 20-25 minutes, or until cauliflower is tender and golden brown.
5. Serve hot.

Nutritional Information (per serving):
- Calories: 70
- Protein: 3g
- Fat: 5g
- Carbohydrates: 6g
- Fiber: 3g

Edamame with Sea Salt

Total Time: 10 minutes
Number of Servings: 4

Ingredients:
- 2 cups frozen edamame (in pods)
- Sea salt to taste

Directions:
1. Bring a pot of water to a boil. Add frozen edamame pods and cook for 5-7 minutes, or until edamame is tender.
2. Drain edamame and transfer to a serving bowl.
3. Sprinkle with sea salt to taste.
4. Serve hot or at room temperature.

Nutritional Information (per serving):
- Calories: 100
- Protein: 9g
- Fat: 3g
- Carbohydrates: 8g
- Fiber: 5g

Carrot and Hummus Snack

Total Time: 10 minutes
Number of Servings: 2

Ingredients:
- 2 large carrots, peeled and cut into sticks
- 1/2 cup hummus

Directions:
1. Arrange carrot sticks on a serving plate.
2. Serve with hummus for dipping.

Nutritional Information (per serving):
- Calories: 100
- Protein: 4g
- Fat: 5g
- Carbohydrates: 12g
- Fiber: 6g

Baked Zucchini Chips

Total Time: 30 minutes
Number of Servings: 4

Ingredients:
- 2 medium zucchinis, thinly sliced
- 2 tablespoons olive oil
- 1/4 cup grated Parmesan cheese
- 1 teaspoon garlic powder
- Salt and pepper to taste

Directions:
1. Preheat the oven to 425°F (220°C).
2. In a large bowl, toss zucchini slices with olive oil, grated Parmesan cheese, garlic powder, salt, and pepper until evenly coated.

3. Arrange zucchini slices in a single layer on a baking sheet lined with parchment paper.
4. Bake in the preheated oven for 20-25 minutes, flipping halfway through, or until zucchini chips are crispy and golden brown.
5. Serve hot or at room temperature.

Nutritional Information (per serving):
- Calories: 80
- Protein: 3g
- Fat: 6g
- Carbohydrates: 5g
- Fiber: 2g

Roasted Red Pepper Hummus with Veggie Sticks

Total Time: 15 minutes
Number of Servings: 4

Ingredients:
- 1 cup roasted red peppers (from a jar), drained
- 1 can (15 oz) chickpeas, drained and rinsed
- 2 tablespoons tahini
- 2 tablespoons lemon juice
- 1 clove garlic
- 2 tablespoons olive oil
- Salt and pepper to taste
- Assorted vegetable sticks (carrots, celery, bell peppers) for serving

Directions:
1. In a food processor, combine roasted red peppers, chickpeas, tahini, lemon juice, garlic, olive oil, salt, and pepper.
2. Blend until smooth and creamy, scraping down the sides of the bowl as needed.
3. Transfer hummus to a serving bowl.
4. Serve with assorted vegetable sticks for dipping.

Nutritional Information (per serving):
- Calories: 120
- Protein: 4g
- Fat: 7g
- Carbohydrates: 12g
- Fiber: 4g

Spinach and Kale Chips

Total Time: 25 minutes
Number of Servings: 4

Ingredients:
- 2 cups fresh spinach leaves
- 2 cups fresh kale leaves, stems removed
- 1 tablespoon olive oil
- Salt and pepper to taste

Directions:
1. Preheat the oven to 350°F (175°C).
2. In a large bowl, toss spinach and kale leaves with olive oil, salt, and pepper until evenly coated.
3. Spread spinach and kale leaves in a single layer on a baking sheet lined with parchment paper.
4. Bake in the preheated oven for 15-20 minutes, or until spinach and kale chips are crispy.
5. Serve immediately.

Nutritional Information (per serving):
- Calories: 30
- Protein: 2g
- Fat: 2g
- Carbohydrates: 3g
- Fiber: 2g

Stuffed Mini Bell Peppers with Quinoa

Total Time: 35 minutes
Number of Servings: 4

Ingredients:
- 8 mini bell peppers, halved and seeded
- 1 cup cooked quinoa
- 1/2 cup black beans, drained and rinsed
- 1/4 cup diced tomatoes
- 1/4 cup diced red onion
- 1/4 cup shredded cheddar cheese
- 1 teaspoon chili powder
- Salt and pepper to taste
- Chopped fresh cilantro for garnish (optional)

Directions:

1. Preheat the oven to 375°F (190°C).
2. In a large bowl, combine cooked quinoa, black beans, diced tomatoes, diced red onion, shredded cheddar cheese, chili powder, salt, and pepper.
3. Spoon the quinoa mixture into each halved mini bell pepper.
4. Place stuffed mini bell peppers on a baking sheet lined with parchment paper.
5. Bake in the preheated oven for 15-20 minutes, or until peppers are tender and filling is heated through.
6. Garnish with chopped fresh cilantro if desired before serving.

Nutritional Information (per serving):

- Calories: 150
- Protein: 6g
- Fat: 5g
- Carbohydrates: 20g
- Fiber: 5g

Dessert

Greek Yogurt with Honey and Almonds

Total Time: 5 minutes
Number of Servings: 2

Ingredients:
- 1 cup Greek yogurt
- 2 tablespoons honey
- 2 tablespoons sliced almonds

Directions:
1. Divide Greek yogurt evenly into serving bowls.
2. Drizzle honey over the yogurt.
3. Sprinkle sliced almonds on top.
4. Serve immediately.

Nutritional Information (per serving):
- Calories: 200
- Protein: 18g
- Fat: 8g
- Carbohydrates: 15g
- Fiber: 1g

Baked Apples with Cinnamon and Walnuts

Total Time: 40 minutes
Number of Servings: 4

Ingredients:
- 4 apples, cored
- 2 tablespoons chopped walnuts
- 1 tablespoon honey
- 1 teaspoon cinnamon

Directions:
1. Preheat the oven to 375°F (190°C).
2. Place cored apples in a baking dish.
3. In a small bowl, mix together chopped walnuts, honey, and cinnamon.
4. Stuff each apple with the walnut mixture.
5. Bake in the preheated oven for 30-35 minutes, or until apples are tender.
6. Serve hot.

Nutritional Information (per serving):
- Calories: 150
- Protein: 2g
- Fat: 4g
- Carbohydrates: 30g
- Fiber: 5g

Chia Seed Pudding with Berries

Total Time: 4 hours 5 minutes
Number of Servings: 2

Ingredients:
- 1/4 cup chia seeds
- 1 cup almond milk (or milk of your choice)
- 1 tablespoon honey (optional)
- 1/2 cup mixed berries (such as strawberries, blueberries, raspberries)

Directions:
1. In a bowl, mix chia seeds, almond milk, and honey (if using).
2. Cover and refrigerate for at least 4 hours or overnight, until thickened.
3. Stir the chia pudding to redistribute the seeds.
4. Divide the pudding into serving bowls.
5. Top with mixed berries before serving.

Nutritional Information (per serving):
- Calories: 150
- Protein: 5g
- Fat: 7g
- Carbohydrates: 20g
- Fiber: 10g

Dark Chocolate Covered Strawberries

Total Time: 20 minutes
Number of Servings: 4

Ingredients:
- 8 large strawberries, washed and dried
- 2 ounces dark chocolate, chopped

Directions:
1. Line a baking sheet with parchment paper.

2. In a microwave-safe bowl, melt the dark chocolate in 30-second intervals, stirring in between until smooth.
3. Dip each strawberry into the melted chocolate, letting any excess drip off.
4. Place the chocolate-covered strawberries on the prepared baking sheet.
5. Refrigerate for 10-15 minutes, or until the chocolate is set.
6. Serve chilled.

Nutritional Information (per serving):
- Calories: 60
- Protein: 1g
- Fat: 4g
- Carbohydrates: 8g
- Fiber: 2g

Almond Flour Cookies with Dark Chocolate Chips

Total Time: 25 minutes
Number of Servings: 12

Ingredients:
- 1 cup almond flour
- 1/4 cup coconut oil, melted
- 1/4 cup honey
- 1 egg
- 1/2 teaspoon vanilla extract
- 1/4 teaspoon baking soda
- Pinch of salt
- 1/4 cup dark chocolate chips

Directions:
1. Preheat the oven to 350°F (175°C). Line a baking sheet with parchment paper.
2. In a bowl, mix together almond flour, melted coconut oil, honey, egg, vanilla extract, baking soda, and salt until well combined.
3. Fold in dark chocolate chips.
4. Drop tablespoonfuls of dough onto the prepared baking sheet, leaving space between each cookie.
5. Flatten each cookie slightly with the back of a spoon.
6. Bake in the preheated oven for 10-12 minutes, or until edges are golden brown.
7. Let the cookies cool on the baking sheet for 5 minutes before transferring to a wire rack to cool completely.

Nutritional Information (per serving):
- Calories: 120
- Protein: 2g

- Fat: 9g
- Carbohydrates: 9g
- Fiber: 1g

Berry Sorbet with Fresh Mint

Total Time: 3 hours 5 minutes
Number of Servings: 4

Ingredients:
- 2 cups mixed berries (such as strawberries, blueberries, raspberries)
- 1 tablespoon honey (optional)
- Fresh mint leaves for garnish

Directions:
1. Place mixed berries in a blender or food processor.
2. Add honey (if using).
3. Blend until smooth.
4. Pour the mixture into a shallow dish and freeze for 2-3 hours, stirring occasionally, until firm but scoopable.
5. Scoop the sorbet into serving bowls.
6. Garnish with fresh mint leaves before serving.

Nutritional Information (per serving):
- Calories: 50
- Protein: 1g
- Fat: 0g
- Carbohydrates: 12g
- Fiber: 4g

Apple and Oat Crumble

Total Time: 45 minutes
Number of Servings: 6

Ingredients:
- 4 apples, peeled, cored, and sliced
- 1 tablespoon lemon juice
- 1/4 cup honey
- 1 teaspoon cinnamon
- 1 cup rolled oats
- 1/4 cup almond flour
- 1/4 cup chopped walnuts
- 2 tablespoons coconut oil, melted

Directions:
1. Preheat the oven to 350°F (175°C). Grease a baking dish with coconut oil.
2. In a bowl, toss apple slices with lemon juice, honey, and cinnamon until evenly coated. Transfer to the prepared baking dish.
3. In another bowl, combine rolled oats, almond flour, chopped walnuts, and melted coconut oil. Mix until crumbly.
4. Sprinkle the oat mixture over the apples in the baking dish.
5. Bake in the preheated oven for 30-35 minutes, or until the topping is golden brown and the apples are tender.
6. Serve warm.

Nutritional Information (per serving):
- Calories: 200
- Protein: 3g
- Fat: 8g
- Carbohydrates: 30g
- Fiber: 5g

Banana and Oatmeal Cookies

Total Time: 20 minutes
Number of Servings: 12

Ingredients:
- 2 ripe bananas, mashed
- 1 cup rolled oats
- 1/4 cup chopped nuts (such as walnuts or almonds)
- 1/4 cup dried fruit (such as raisins or cranberries)
- 1/4 teaspoon cinnamon
- Pinch of salt

Directions:
1. Preheat the oven to 350°F (175°C). Line a baking sheet with parchment paper.
2. In a bowl, combine mashed bananas, rolled oats, chopped nuts, dried fruit, cinnamon, and salt. Mix until well combined.
3. Drop tablespoonfuls of dough onto the prepared baking sheet, leaving space between each cookie.
4. Flatten each cookie slightly with the back of a spoon.
5. Bake in the preheated oven for 15-18 minutes, or until golden brown.
6. Let the cookies cool on the baking sheet for 5 minutes before transferring to a wire rack to cool completely.

Nutritional Information (per serving):
- Calories: 70
- Protein: 2g
- Fat: 2g
- Carbohydrates: 12g
- Fiber: 2g

Blueberry and Almond Smoothie Bowl

Total Time: 5 minutes
Number of Servings: 1

Ingredients:
- 1 frozen banana
- 1/2 cup frozen blueberries
- 1/2 cup almond milk
- 1 tablespoon almond butter
- 1 tablespoon chia seeds
- 1 tablespoon sliced almonds
- Fresh blueberries for garnish

Directions:
1. In a blender, combine frozen banana, frozen blueberries, almond milk, almond butter, and chia seeds. Blend until smooth.
2. Pour the smoothie into a bowl.
3. Top with sliced almonds and fresh blueberries.
4. Serve immediately.

Nutritional Information (per serving):
- Calories: 350
- Protein: 9g
- Fat: 15g
- Carbohydrates: 45g
- Fiber: 10g

Quinoa and Coconut Pudding

Total Time: 30 minutes (plus chilling time)
Number of Servings: 4

Ingredients:
- 1/2 cup quinoa
- 1 can (14 oz) coconut milk

- 1/4 cup honey or maple syrup
- 1 teaspoon vanilla extract
- Pinch of salt
- Shredded coconut and fresh berries for garnish (optional)

Directions:
1. Rinse quinoa under cold water in a fine mesh sieve.
2. In a saucepan, combine rinsed quinoa, coconut milk, honey or maple syrup, vanilla extract, and a pinch of salt.
3. Bring the mixture to a boil over medium heat, then reduce the heat to low and simmer for 15-20 minutes, stirring occasionally, until the quinoa is cooked and the mixture has thickened.
4. Remove the saucepan from the heat and let the pudding cool slightly.
5. Transfer the pudding to serving bowls or glasses and refrigerate for at least 2 hours, or until chilled and set.
6. Garnish with shredded coconut and fresh berries before serving, if desired.

Nutritional Information (per serving):
- Calories: 250
- Protein: 5g
- Fat: 15g
- Carbohydrates: 25g
- Fiber: 2g

Smoothie

Spinach and Pineapple Smoothie

Total Time: 5 minutes
Number of Servings: 1

Ingredients:
- 1 cup fresh spinach leaves
- 1/2 cup frozen pineapple chunks
- 1/2 banana
- 1/2 cup almond milk
- 1/4 cup Greek yogurt
- Honey or maple syrup to taste (optional)
- Ice cubes (optional)

Directions:
1. Place all ingredients in a blender.
2. Blend until smooth and creamy.
3. If desired, add honey or maple syrup to sweeten, and ice cubes for a colder smoothie.
4. Pour into a glass and serve immediately.

Nutritional Information (per serving):
- Calories: 150
- Protein: 6g
- Fat: 3g
- Carbohydrates: 30g
- Fiber: 4g

Berry and Flaxseed Smoothie

Total Time: 5 minutes
Number of Servings: 1

Ingredients:
- 1/2 cup mixed berries (such as strawberries, blueberries, raspberries)
- 1/2 banana
- 1 tablespoon ground flaxseeds
- 1/2 cup almond milk
- 1/4 cup Greek yogurt
- Honey or maple syrup to taste (optional)
- Ice cubes (optional)

Directions:

1. Place all ingredients in a blender.
2. Blend until smooth and creamy.
3. If desired, add honey or maple syrup to sweeten, and ice cubes for a colder smoothie.
4. Pour into a glass and serve immediately.

Nutritional Information (per serving):

- Calories: 180
- Protein: 6g
- Fat: 5g
- Carbohydrates: 30g
- Fiber: 7g

Avocado and Banana Smoothie

Total Time: 5 minutes
Number of Servings: 1

Ingredients:

- 1/2 ripe avocado
- 1/2 banana
- 1 tablespoon honey or maple syrup
- 1/2 cup almond milk
- 1/4 cup Greek yogurt
- Ice cubes (optional)

Directions:

1. Scoop out the avocado flesh and place it in a blender.
2. Add banana, honey or maple syrup, almond milk, Greek yogurt, and ice cubes.
3. Blend until smooth and creamy.
4. Pour into a glass and serve immediately.

Nutritional Information (per serving):

- Calories: 250
- Protein: 7g
- Fat: 12g
- Carbohydrates: 30g
- Fiber: 7g

Green Tea and Mango Smoothie

Total Time: 5 minutes
Number of Servings: 1

Ingredients:
- 1/2 cup brewed green tea, cooled
- 1/2 cup frozen mango chunks
- 1/2 banana
- 1 tablespoon honey or maple syrup
- 1/4 cup Greek yogurt
- Ice cubes (optional)

Directions:
1. In a blender, combine brewed green tea, frozen mango chunks, banana, honey or maple syrup, Greek yogurt, and ice cubes.
2. Blend until smooth and creamy.
3. Pour into a glass and serve immediately.

Nutritional Information (per serving):
- Calories: 200
- Protein: 6g
- Fat: 2g
- Carbohydrates: 40g
- Fiber: 5g

Kale and Apple Smoothie

Total Time: 5 minutes
Number of Servings: 1

Ingredients:
- 1 cup chopped kale leaves
- 1/2 apple, cored and chopped
- 1/2 banana
- 1 tablespoon almond butter
- 1/2 cup almond milk
- 1/4 cup Greek yogurt
- Honey or maple syrup to taste (optional)
- Ice cubes (optional)

Directions:
1. Place all ingredients in a blender.

2. Blend until smooth and creamy.
3. If desired, add honey or maple syrup to sweeten, and ice cubes for a colder smoothie.
4. Pour into a glass and serve immediately.

Nutritional Information (per serving):
- Calories: 220
- Protein: 8g
- Fat: 8g
- Carbohydrates: 30g
- Fiber: 6g

Almond Butter and Banana Smoothie

Total Time: 5 minutes
Number of Servings: 1

Ingredients:
- 1 tablespoon almond butter
- 1/2 banana
- 1/2 cup almond milk
- 1/4 cup Greek yogurt
- 1 teaspoon honey or maple syrup
- Ice cubes (optional)

Directions:
1. Place almond butter, banana, almond milk, Greek yogurt, honey or maple syrup, and ice cubes in a blender.
2. Blend until smooth and creamy.
3. Pour into a glass and serve immediately.

Nutritional Information (per serving):
- Calories: 250
- Protein: 8g
- Fat: 14g
- Carbohydrates: 30g
- Fiber: 5g

Mixed Berry and Chia Seed Smoothie

Total Time: 5 minutes
Number of Servings: 1

Ingredients:
- 1/2 cup mixed berries (such as strawberries, blueberries, raspberries)
- 1/2 banana
- 1 tablespoon chia seeds
- 1/2 cup almond milk
- 1/4 cup Greek yogurt
- Honey or maple syrup to taste (optional)
- Ice cubes (optional)

Directions:
1. Place all ingredients in a blender.
2. Blend until smooth and creamy.
3. If desired, add honey or maple syrup to sweeten, and ice cubes for a colder smoothie.
4. Pour into a glass and serve immediately.

Nutritional Information (per serving):
- Calories: 200
- Protein: 6g
- Fat: 5g
- Carbohydrates: 30g
- Fiber: 8g

Spinach and Avocado Smoothie

Total Time: 5 minutes
Number of Servings: 1

Ingredients:
- 1 cup fresh spinach leaves
- 1/4 avocado
- 1/2 banana
- 1/2 cup almond milk
- 1/4 cup Greek yogurt
- Honey or maple syrup to taste (optional)
- Ice cubes (optional)

Directions:
1. Place all ingredients in a blender.

2. Blend until smooth and creamy.
3. If desired, add honey or maple syrup to sweeten, and ice cubes for a colder smoothie.
4. Pour into a glass and serve immediately.

Nutritional Information (per serving):
- Calories: 180
- Protein: 6g
- Fat: 8g
- Carbohydrates: 25g
- Fiber: 6g

Pineapple and Coconut Smoothie

Total Time: 5 minutes
Number of Servings: 1

Ingredients:
- 1/2 cup frozen pineapple chunks
- 1/2 banana
- 1/2 cup coconut milk
- 1/4 cup Greek yogurt
- Honey or maple syrup to taste (optional)
- Ice cubes (optional)

Directions:
1. Place all ingredients in a blender.
2. Blend until smooth and creamy.
3. If desired, add honey or maple syrup to sweeten, and ice cubes for a colder smoothie.
4. Pour into a glass and serve immediately.

Nutritional Information (per serving):
- Calories: 220
- Protein: 6g
- Fat: 10g
- Carbohydrates: 30g
- Fiber: 5g

Blueberry and Almond Milk Smoothie

Total Time: 5 minutes
Number of Servings: 1

Ingredients:
- 1/2 cup blueberries
- 1/2 banana
- 1/2 cup almond milk
- 1/4 cup Greek yogurt
- 1 tablespoon almond butter
- Honey or maple syrup to taste (optional)
- Ice cubes (optional)

Directions:
1. Place all ingredients in a blender.
2. Blend until smooth and creamy.
3. If desired, add honey or maple syrup to sweeten, and ice cubes for a colder smoothie.
4. Pour into a glass and serve immediately.

Nutritional Information (per serving):
- Calories: 200
- Protein: 7g
- Fat: 8g
- Carbohydrates: 30g
- Fiber: 6g

14-Day Meal Plan

Day 1:
- **Breakfast:** Spinach and Pineapple Smoothie
- **Lunch:** Grilled Chicken and Quinoa Salad with Lemon Dressing
- **Dinner:** Baked Salmon with Asparagus and Quinoa

Day 2:
- **Breakfast:** Berry and Flaxseed Smoothie
- **Lunch:** Lentil and Vegetable Soup
- **Dinner:** Vegetable Stir-Fry with Brown Rice

Day 3:
- **Breakfast:** Avocado and Banana Smoothie
- **Lunch:** Spinach and Strawberry Salad with Walnuts
- **Dinner:** Lentil Shepherd's Pie with Sweet Potato Topping

Day 4:
- **Breakfast:** Green Tea and Mango Smoothie
- **Lunch:** Black Bean and Corn Salad with Lime Dressing
- **Dinner:** Grilled Chicken with Roasted Vegetables

Day 5:
- **Breakfast:** Kale and Apple Smoothie
- **Lunch:** Tuna and Avocado Salad on Whole Grain Crackers
- **Dinner:** Chickpea and Cauliflower Curry with Brown Rice

Day 6:
- **Breakfast:** Almond Butter and Banana Smoothie
- **Lunch:** Mediterranean Quinoa Salad with Olives and Feta
- **Dinner:** Stuffed Eggplant with Quinoa and Vegetables

Day 7:
- **Breakfast:** Mixed Berry and Chia Seed Smoothie
- **Lunch:** Lentil and Sweet Potato Stew
- **Dinner:** Grilled Shrimp Skewers with Quinoa Salad

Day 8:
- **Breakfast:** Spinach and Avocado Smoothie
- **Lunch:** Roasted Butternut Squash Soup
- **Dinner:** Baked Cod with Garlic and Lemon

Day 9:
- **Breakfast:** Pineapple and Coconut Smoothie
- **Lunch:** Chickpea and Spinach Curry
- **Dinner:** Turkey Meatballs with Whole Grain Spaghetti

Day 10:
- **Breakfast:** Blueberry and Almond Milk Smoothie
- **Lunch:** Greek Salad with Quinoa
- **Dinner:** Grilled Tofu with Quinoa and Steamed Broccoli

Day 11:
- **Breakfast:** Berry Sorbet with Fresh Mint
- **Lunch:** Lentil Soup with Carrots and Celery
- **Dinner:** Baked Tilapia with Herbs and Brown Rice

Day 12:
- **Breakfast:** Quinoa and Coconut Pudding
- **Lunch:** Spinach and Kale Salad with Sunflower Seeds
- **Dinner:** Turkey and Vegetable Stir-Fry

Day 13:
- **Breakfast:** Flaxseed and Banana Smoothie
- **Lunch:** Tomato Basil Soup
- **Dinner:** Mediterranean Baked Chicken with Olives and Tomatoes

Day 14:
- **Breakfast:** Chia Seed Pudding with Berries
- **Lunch:** Brown Rice and Edamame Salad
- **Dinner:** Vegetable Stir-Fry with Brown Rice

Conclusion

In the journey towards optimal health, the significance of a prostate-healthy diet cannot be overstated. Throughout this comprehensive guide, we've delved into the intricate relationship between nutrition and prostate health, providing insights, recipes, and strategies tailored specifically for men over 40. Prostate cancer, a condition affecting millions of men worldwide, often underscores the necessity of proactive dietary choices. Through understanding the role of diet in prostate health, we've uncovered how certain foods can either promote or hinder prostate wellness. Key nutrients, antioxidants, and phytochemicals found abundantly in fruits, vegetables, whole grains, lean proteins, and healthy fats have emerged as pillars of a prostate-healthy diet. Conversely, processed foods, excessive red meat consumption, and saturated fats have been linked to increased prostate cancer risk.

By embracing a diet rich in colorful fruits, leafy greens, whole grains, and lean proteins, men over 40 can empower themselves in the fight against prostate cancer. These dietary choices not only contribute to prostate health but also support overall well-being, bolstering immune function, cardiovascular health, and energy levels. Embarking on the path to a prostate-healthy diet involves more than just short-term adjustments—it necessitates a commitment to long-term lifestyle changes. While the prospect of altering dietary habits may seem daunting, the rewards far outweigh the challenges. By viewing dietary modifications as an investment in one's health and longevity, individuals can cultivate sustainable habits that endure beyond the confines of this guide. Small, incremental changes can yield profound results over time. Whether it's swapping processed snacks for nutrient-dense alternatives, incorporating more plant-based meals into one's diet, or experimenting with new recipes, every step towards a prostate-healthy lifestyle is a step towards vitality and resilience.

As we conclude this journey through the intricacies of a prostate-healthy diet, it's essential to remember that the power to transform our health lies within each of us. By harnessing the healing potential of wholesome foods and embracing a lifestyle rooted in balance and moderation, men over 40 can cultivate resilience in the face of prostate cancer and other chronic illnesses. Let us approach each meal as an opportunity to nourish our bodies, fuel our vitality, and honor the profound connection between nutrition and well-being. Together, let us embark on this journey towards vibrant health and longevity, armed with knowledge, determination, and the unwavering belief in our ability to thrive.
In the pursuit of optimal health, may we find strength in the choices we make, the meals we savor, and the journey we undertake towards a future brimming with vitality, purpose, and abundant well-being.